THE STORY OF AQUALEAD

A New Healing Energy for a New Earth

SABINE BLAIS

SILGEROND PRESS

The Story of Aqualead

A New Healing Energy for a New Earth

This book is a reference work based on the author's educational, teaching and practical experience. The information contained herein is in no way to be considered as a substitute for consultation with a duly licensed physician.

ISBN 978-0-9936322-0-4

Sabine Blais

Published by
Silgerond Press
Gatineau, Québec, Canada
www.silgerond.blogspot.com
sabine.ggr@gmail.com

Printed and bound in Canada

Cover Illustration: Sabine Blais
Graphic Design: Gregory Banks
Editing: Sigrid Macdonald

Library and Archives Canada Cataloguing in Publication

Blais, Sabine, 1971 –
The Story of Aqualead / Sabine Blais.

"The beauty of Elves resides in their harmony with nature and their love of trees."

- *Sabine Blais*

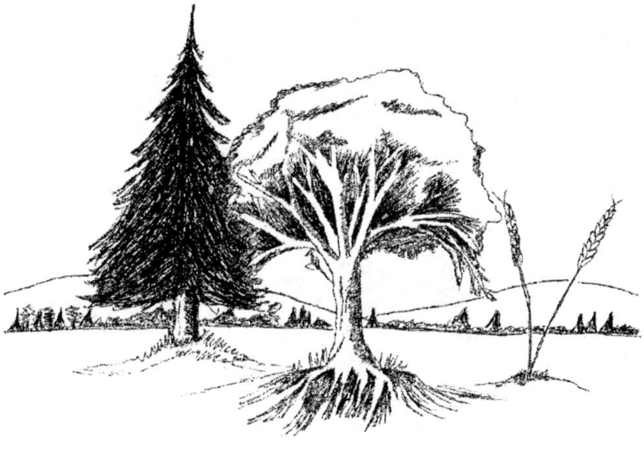

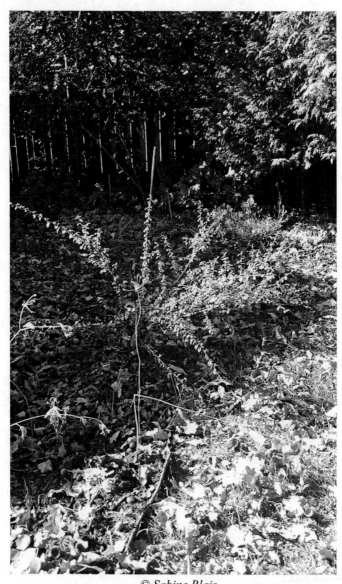

© *Sabine Blais*

Table of Contents

TABLE OF ILLUSTRATIONS

DEDICATION

This book is dedicated to Mother Earth, to all the trees and to all the animals that grace the world with their presence. This work is also dedicated to the forces of nature and the four elements, which move everything around us in the perpetual cycle of transformation and renewal. To the guardians of the Earth, who have watched over the planet and all its life forms over millions of years, and who have witnessed the birth of mankind and all its changes.

ACKNOWLEGMENTS

I am most grateful to all the growing Aqualead communities worldwide for their ongoing support, insights and persistent hard work with this new healing energy. I am also grateful to the amazing and supportive students I have had the honour of working with, from the very beginning of this journey with Aqualead. The trust, confidence and enthusiasm my friends demonstrated for Aqualead in Argentina, when it first came out, was a confirmation to me that this was truly happening, and was just *meant to be.* I had no doubt from the beginning, and I am thankful for the faith and trust (and patience) of others throughout the development of Aqualead, over the recent years.

I extend my infinite gratitude to my friend Andrés Gosis in Buenos Aires, who was the first person to come in contact with the energy of Aqualead after it was channelled. He received the first healing session and Aqualead attunement.

I also extend my deepest gratitude to Aqualead Masters Claudio Fafian, Ana Zanuy, Jime del Hierro and Maria Magdalena Vivas Mansilla in Buenos Aires (Capital) for their hard work; to Marian Gillyatt in the province of Bs. As., Roberto Camino, Lorena Muiños and Claudia Córdoba for their ongoing friendship and caring presence. To Patricio Simini and Christine Johnson in Bariloche (southern Argentina) for their unfailing support, and to my dear friends Liliana Sanchez de Ron, Ana Maria Sequalino, Marisa Ferrer, Federico Gonzalez, Alfonsina

D'Attellis, Erica Agüero and Mirian Ana Spinelli in Rosario, Santa Fé; to Sandra Paquez and Dario Veron in the sierras of Capilla del Monte, Cordoba, who opened their doors to us at their healing centre in the mountains; as well as to Marcela Barrios from Cordoba City.

I take this opportunity to thank my Kung Fu teacher in Belgrano and others in Buenos Aires, for the many challenges they have brought me.

In Canada, I am thankful to my mother Josée Gaspard Blais, my Reiki Master Maria Trumbach in Ottawa and to my great friend and Aqualead Master Celeste Grenon in Vancouver, B.C., for their immense support.

I also thank my great friends Maria Shanko and Vigdis Steinthorsdóttir in Reykjavik, Iceland, and Sara Ramirez in New Jersey, United States; also Carlos Villa Guzman and Silvia Medina in Mexico and Mauricio Bentos and Sabrina Zapata in Uruguay for playing crucial roles in the spread of Aqualead worldwide. All of these amazing people served as an inspiration for writing this book.

I would like to extend my immense gratitude to my ever-present guides, the old and wise elemental beings that surround me, and to their constant presence I feel when I am working with or teaching Aqualead. I thank my masters from afar for having sent me this gift, and for bringing out the master in me. We are all one.

PREFACE

This book is a memoir of the journey and development of Aqualead during the first five years of its presence, from the beginning. Despite its short history, many changes, developments and transformations have occurred at the personal, emotional and environmental levels with the presence and use of Aqualead. These changes were deeply felt by many of us who have been working diligently with this new energy for some years. For some people, like myself, the arrival of Aqualead marked a significant turning point in their life.

Even though these memoirs are a compilation of my experiences and observations, after serving as a channel for Aqualead and teaching it in different parts of the world, I am not writing these pages alone. Without the hundreds of Aqualead practitioners and Masters worldwide, and the growing interest and support for Aqualead, I would not be undertaking the writing of this book. I write this book with all of them in mind, the global Aqualead community, whose lives and hearts were touched by Aqualead, and who share the feeling of commuting with a part of them that was thought to be forgotten. It is that feeling of unity and the desire for change which draws many people towards learning Aqualead, and it is that feeling I wish to convey to you, the reader, as you go through these pages.

Throughout the book I will use the first person, but it is by no means my intention to draw all the credit and glory upon myself throughout this huge effort. The first person is used rather because at the very beginning, there was no else who had made contact with this energy before, and I was the only person who held these memories and experiences of how Aqualead made its way into this troubled world in such a timely fashion. I am speaking on behalf of a strong and proud community of healers; some with a certain amount of previous experience using healing energy, others without, but who share the same desire: to see this planet heal, to see nature restored and to make this world a safer and better place for all living creatures.

This book is intended as a general overview of what Aqualead is, where it came from, its purpose and how it came about. It was clear to me from the beginning that this book needed to be accessible to *everyone*, regardless of previous experience, knowledge of Aqualead or background. This book is not a training manual, reserved only for those learning Aqualead, nor is it only for Aqualead practitioners and Masters. This publication is not to be used in Aqualead classes or seminars as a part of the Aqualead Program, in order to learn the modality. Instead, anyone and everyone can read this book, and hopefully enjoy the experience of seeing the world from the perspective of an environmental healer, working with new tools.

The introduction is where all the information about the Aqualead modality itself is explained and described. Some additional information is provided as well, in order to make it easier for the inexperienced reader to understand some terms or concepts (such as an *attunement* and *elemental being*). The nine chapters that follow consist of my account of how Aqualead appeared and was channelled, and my experience working with this new energy that was still unknown at the time. Some further reflections follow in the remaining chapters, about the practice of Aqualead and the essential relationship that binds the Aqualead practitioner and Master to the elements of nature and its inhabitants. Aqualead reminds us that the *outdoors* and n*ature* are not places that are remote or far away but rather immediately around us.

I took great care throughout the writing of this book to maintain the integrity of the modality and its principles of freedom from the material world. I had a strong and deep feeling that this book needed to be produced here in Canada, in order for Aqualead to make its formal appearance in the world, and for the energy to express itself. After five years of existence in this world and dimension, this encounter was now due to occur. It is my hope that the publication of this book will not alter the message behind this elemental energy, and its freedom from monetary obligations. Rather, I see this book as a helpful vehicle to spread the information and knowledge of this new healing system to every corner of the world. The more people who know about the existence of Aqualead, the more the good news is shared with others.

It is also my hope that readers will get a better grasp, after reading these pages, of the new, subtle energies that have recently entered this world, and that despite the damage done to this planet in so little time, *we are being helped.* Aqualead's recent arrival in our world has already signalled this help we are receiving, as we now have new tools that enable us to do more for this planet, in order to assist it in regaining its balance and original state of purity.

May this gift we have received and discovered through Aqualead reach you, the readers of the *Story of Aqualead: A New Healing Energy for a New Earth.* May you reconnect, by reading this book, with the element that lies within us, in every cell: *water.* Perhaps by reading this publication and learning more about Aqualead, you will also feel compelled to be a part of this magical elemental energy, and become a part of this new family.

Sabine Blais
August 8th, 2013

INTRODUCTION

The subject of Aqualead and the repercussions it has on the outside world is a very vast subject. Before readers undertake reading the chapters of this book, I felt necessary, through this introduction, to present an overview of what Aqualead is, what it consists of and the general training program that has been established. Hence, this section will be greatly valuable to assist readers in better understanding certain terms, and feel more comfortable with the context and the subject of the book. This initial orientation for those unfamiliar with Aqualead and energy work is, in my opinion, essential in order to better grasp the narration in this book.

The book is divided into three parts. The first part discuses my personal story of moving to Argentina and discovering Aqualead while living in Buenos Aires. The chapters also reveal some of my travels and encounters I have made with other healers, as I developed this new modality. The second part of the book discusses the general practices related to Aqualead, and my personal account and observations of working with it, as well as with other practitioners and Masters. The third part is focused on nature itself, and how Aqualead can help assist and rebalance the Earth from various angles; for instance, through healing the oceans, protecting forests, and more awareness of animals. Two appendices were added to this book; Appendix I contains the

Aqualead principles, which reflect the general philosophy behind the practice of Aqualead. Appendix II is a compilation of 12 tips for everyone to follow in order to help the Earth become greener and healthier.

I have added below some general information about Aqualead, which explains what this energy is. This is only a general overview, and is aimed at preparing and helping inexperienced readers to enter the subject of this book and follow it throughout the chapters. I have also included a brief explanation of elemental beings, which is a subject that appears frequently in the realm of Aqualead. This way the readers, I hope, will not feel lost or left behind as they go through the pages of this book.

i. A general description

Aqualead is a new energy that heals water in living beings and in the environment. The name has the word *aqua* attached to it, which is reminiscent of water, however, it is not a source of water, nor is it associated with any aquatic sport, or activity done under water. This new healing energy was channelled in downtown Buenos Aires, Argentina, on August 30th, 2008. Aqualead is an energy that has a strong affinity with water, and has a very purifying effect on the environment and living organisms. However, one who starts learning Aqualead soon realizes that healing water is only the beginning of what Aqualead is able to do, as the energy can accomplish much more than just decontaminate water.

It is a subtle energy sent to us from a different part of the universe. The energy of Aqualead is an *elemental energy*, and has a very natural yet powerful feel to it. It creates a powerful connection to the elements of nature, nature beings and the Earth itself. Aqualead constitutes a balance, being a very high frequency energy related to the angelic realm, yet very grounding and focused on healing and rebalancing nature. The energy is wise and intelligent, and guides the practitioner or Master in their practice of the energy and in their daily lives. The term *Aqualead* is applied to designate the energy itself, as well as the modality or healing system by the same name. Aqualead energy is practised or applied through the hands over a person or living being. It can also be sent remotely, in order to perform healing at a distance.

The channelling process of Aqualead was completely unexpected and, as opposed to what some may assume, I was not in any state of trance or deep meditation when it occurred. Being a healing energy, Aqualead is only used to produce positive results or to create a healing effect on a certain situation. Aqualead is not negative, nor can it be used for negative purposes. It is rather an angelic ray of energy, of a very high vibration, and at the beginning of the channelling process, an angel was present with me. The angel's name was Ariel, an angel I was already familiar with through previous energy work with angels. After doing some research, I discovered that angel Ariel is the angel that oversees the Earth and is closely related to the element of water, which I did not really know at the time of the channelling. The origin of Aqualead is not of this world. It arrived here from another part of the universe; aside from having a higher frequency of energy than our own, Aqualead is also of a higher dimension. This is a new energy arriving to us from another world; and by this energy being now present among us, it is helping bring this world into an evolutionary shift towards a higher dimension.

The feel of Aqualead is quite strong, and for those who are already acquainted with Reiki and beginning to use Aqualead, the difference between the two energies is obvious. Aqualead has a different personality than Reiki, being a more dynamic, expressive energy that acts very quickly. It should be reminded that Aqualead is *not* Reiki, nor is it a style of Reiki, despite the similarities in their practices; it is a completely distinctive and new energy. Because it is an energy healing modality, Aqualead ranks among the holistic therapies and other energetic healing practices. It could also be compared to an environmental movement, correlated with conservation societies and animal rights groups; Aqualead is deeply rooted within nature, trees, wildlife and natural bodies of water. This healing system is neither a religion nor affiliated with any religious denomination. Despite the fact that an angel was present during the initial channelling phase of Aqualead, it is not a cult to angel Ariel or to any deity. The spirituality in Aqualead does not derive from any religious background but rather through working with a subtle healing energy, bringing Light into the world, and through listening to the universe while paying attention to the guidance it sends us.

ii. The purpose of Aqualead

Aqualead is a therapeutic healing system which is practised by laying of the hands. It can be done on another living being, and can also be practised in self-healing. The initial purpose of Aqualead was to heal water. This does not imply that water should be viewed as a patient with a sickness but rather that the healing performed on water with Aqualead is an act of *decontamination*. Water is inherently pure and innocent in its own natural state. It is a mutable element and can mimic or reflect its surrounding environment. It has the ability to capture and retain information: just like any computer, water can be programmed with various messages, codes or frequencies of energy. The proximity of human cities to bodies of water will cause the water to reflect the general state of mind and emotional state of their inhabitants. Pollution occurs not only at the chemical level but also at the energetic and emotional levels. Aqualead energy has the ability to remove any lower or unwanted energies and clear the water in order to return it back to its original state, in the environment or within a living being. Rivers, lakes and oceans can retain the violence, rage and cruelty generated by human aggression, crimes and wars. The change starts when we reprogram water and replace these lower energies with something more peaceful and positive.

The vast majority of the environmental contamination in the world is due to water becoming contaminated by human activity. Most of the planet's surface is covered with water, and there is always a percentage of water present in the atmosphere, in the form of clouds, mist or rain. However, Aqualead can do far more than just heal water; through the different symbols used, it is able to work through many different aspects of healing, which moves us beyond the scope of water. For instance, the energy of Aqualead is able to facilitate communication between humans and animals, through the use of a certain symbol which enhances a loving and understanding interaction with all creatures. That same function works by enhancing telepathy between the minds of different beings. Another function of Aqualead deals with agriculture and plant growth, enhancing safe, organic and sustainable agriculture.

The healing work can then be specifically focused on trees, plant growth and protecting forests.

As practitioners advance in their Aqualead practice, they can focus their work with Aqualead on a more abstract level, dealing with issues that are not necessarily related to water or nature. With Aqualead, it is possible to dispel negative energy and bring a positive transformation of just about any situation to a higher level of order. It is possible to promote peace and justice with Aqualead, as well as support and facilitate the arts and support the works of artists. We can see here that the practice of Aqualead is a universe in itself and becomes a new challenge for healers who enter and explore this new journey. The practice of Aqualead also paves the way for new alternative forms of energy, and allows one to push the limits of their normal capacities to the next step.

iii. Environmentalism and animal rights

Due to the nature of this energy, the practice of Aqualead focuses on environmental issues, conservation, wildlife preservation and reducing the violence inflicted on animals by humans. At this time, there are rising concerns about current issues, such as the melting of the polar ice caps, the production of genetically-modified foods, global climate changes and the persistent poaching of endangered species. These issues can be specifically addressed with the energy of Aqualead. This is what this energy is here to address, in a most direct and effective way. In these types of situations, a more focused and concentrated healing energy was required; and Aqualead tackles these situations in an almost aggressive, invasive manner. Even better, the healing can be sent remotely at a distance, without being physically present or exposed to any direct danger.

Group healings are particularly effective when dealing with environmental or conservation issues. Healers may opt to meet at a certain location and send energy to the area or water at the same time, in unison. However, this can also be done at a distance, without the healers even being physically at the same location. They can coordinate a time and send Aqualead energy all at the same time, even from different parts of the world. All Aqualead practitioners can send distant healing; this ability is not reserved to a certain level of Aqualead. The healers could send Aqualead in unison to a river or the ocean in order to decontaminate; they can also direct it to a group of people or an organization (such as a corporation) to help raise consciousness about pollution and bring a more positive outcome regarding an environmental issue. The energy can also be sent to a person in order to heal the water in their tissues, thus improving their overall health and well-being.

Aqualead has the characteristic of enhancing one's sensitivity and intuition. In this trend, a higher sensitivity and awareness towards animal life was noticed, as well as the need to respect them. The heightened energy vibration enables people to reach a greater level of awareness, and to feel these changes in their bodies and their habits. After learning Aqualead, it was not uncommon for some people to change their dietary habits, abandoning certain types of foods (such as meat or sugar), or curb certain habits such as drinking coffee, and instead drink more water. Many new Aqualead practitioners have also noted changes in their relationships, and have found themselves severing ties with certain persons, and instead attracting new people and relationships in their lives. This deep transformation was noticed in many people who started learning Aqualead: their overall health increased, a new glow appeared in their faces, and a greater level of joy and personal happiness was achieved. Some people became vegetarian; others deepened their spiritual practices, while other became devoted teachers of the modality and still have many students.

Many Aqualead practitioners and Masters deepen their relationship with nature itself, by retreating or hiking more in the woods and countryside. It seems that Aqualead brings out the *Elf* in some people. For this reason, when embarking in the world of Aqualead, one inevitably becomes closer to nature. Many involved with the energy also become the equivalent of *Environmental activists* or *Animal Rights activists*; however, the necessity for such people in the world is obvious, and Aqualead fully supports them. Then we see how this energy wants to balance all life on Earth and bring this planet to its original state of innocence, and bring a greater justice for all life.

iv. A note about elemental beings

The term *elemental being* returns frequently when discussing Aqualead energy. An elemental being is a nature being, which is commonly found in a natural habitat such as in trees, lakes or mountains. There are many different types of elementals, and they may dwell in different places. The majority of people who are not tuned into higher frequencies cannot see or perceive elemental beings; they appear invisible. It takes a heightened awareness of them and a sharpened perception to see them, hear them and interact with them. However, some people may have spontaneous encounters with them when they least expect it.

Types of elemental beings range from a wide variety of shapes, sizes and cross many different human cultures: for example, Fairies, Elves, Gnomes, Giants, and Trolls. Other types of elemental beings, also referred to as *Fairy Folk,* include Dwarves, Brownies, Kobolds, Pixies, the *Sidhe* and Mermaids. Some elemental beings have *shape shifting* abilities, such as the Giants and certain Fairies, taking the shape of their environment; some may appear as animals, trees, plants or rocks. Depending on their type, elemental beings can range from a height of only three inches tall to several hundred feet high, to the size (and appearance) of a mountain. Gnomes and Fairies are the most well-known elementals, and are often referred to as the *Little People,* in different parts of the Western world. Elves are considered the taller and *wiser* of elementals, averaging the size of a human being. The Elves are more spiritually advanced than other races of elementals.

Some country or culture-specific elementals include the Leprechauns and the *Sidhe* (pronounced *Shee),* which are typical to Ireland. In Argentina, Gnomes are called *Duendes*, or *Abuelitos* (meaning

Little Old Men). Kobolds are common in German folklore, while the knowledge and sightings of Elves are widespread and deeply rooted in Icelandic and Scandinavian cultures. In France and French Canada, Gnomes are known as *Lutins* or *Farfadets*. Besides the typical forests where one is most likely to encounter Fairies, elemental beings can also be seen in mountains, fields, lakes, living underwater, in the ocean and by the seashore. Many elementals in Iceland dwell inside rocks and stones, which gives them an eerie, lifelike appearance. Some of them may opt to reside in human households, and perform house chores around the property, such as the Brownies. There are elemental beings associated with each of the four elements found in nature (fire, air, water and earth). And within each one of us, there is what is known as the *Body Elemental*, with which it is possible to establish communication.

Becoming aware of the presence of such beings allows us to realize how alive and present the forces of nature are around us. The elementals exert their influence over the elements of nature and fulfill their function as guardians and protectors of forests, animals, water and mountains. We see that nature is full of spirit and intelligent life, and that presence, which parallels our own, is to be acknowledged and respected. The energy of Aqualead greatly changes one's energy frequency in order to facilitate the perception of the Fairy People and even communication with them. The elementals are always willing and eager to cooperate with humans, in the common goal of healing the Earth and protecting natural spaces against human destruction. After all, the woods and forests are their home. It seems the added support the energy provides for the elementals is needed, and will hopefully bring positive changes in the realm of nature itself, likely in the most surprising ways.

v. The Aqualead Program

The Aqualead Program is the bulk of the course contents taught to all students, divided in three definite levels. The program is an established and unified guideline, everywhere in the world where Aqualead is taught. The practice and teaching of Aqualead is therefore standardized worldwide, and for this reason I have founded the *International Centre of Aqualead* in 2010. This ensures the continuity, consistency and quality of teaching that students anywhere in the world will receive. It also ensures that the attunement will be performed by Aqualead Masters the exact same way, ensuring that the modality will be transmitted correctly and will continue propagating itself for many years to come. The three levels of Aqualead are as follows:

Aqualead Level I – Healing Water in Living Beings: This level is focused on healing water inside of living organisms, and also includes a component on animal communication. The student is introduced to Aqualead, taught how to give the healing session, learns the first two symbols and how to do the first meditation. The student receives the Aqualead level I attunement, and then practises the healing session and distant healing in the class. *There is no prerequisite for this class.*

Aqualead Level II – Environmental Healing:
This level is focused on environmental healing; it entails healing water all over the planet; dealing with agriculture and plant life; transforming situations, enhancing creativity, and transmuting lower, negative energies into a higher order. The student learns the next three symbols, another meditation, and receives the Aqualead level II attunement. There is a distant healing practice in the class. *Prerequisite: Aqualead level I.*

Aqualead Master (III) – Manifestation:
This level focuses on manifestation and teaching Aqualead; the student learns how to attract and manifest water; new alternative forms of energy; how to send distant healing using crystals; how to teach Aqualead and give the attunements. The student learns the last four symbols and the third meditation; receives the Master level attunement, and then practises giving an attunement. *Prerequisite: Aqualead level II and minimum four months' experience.*

In order to practise Aqualead, the students must receive the *attunement* in the class by a recognized Aqualead Master. The *attunement* is the process in which the Master opens the energy centres (called *chakras*) in the student. This process allows the recipient (the student) to become a channel for the energy, and can later transmit the energy to another person or living thing in a healing session, or can send it at a distance. The attunement is permanent; once you have Aqualead, you have it for life. There is a different attunement at each level of Aqualead.

However, there are no distant classes or attunements in Aqualead; all courses must be done in person with the Master.

There is a minimum wait time between levels of Aqualead. Between the first two levels, there must be a wait time of a minimum of 24 hours. The reason for this is to allow the student to rest after receiving an attunement, and must allow time for the energy to settle in the person's physical body. After receiving an attunement, the person's energy will undergo certain changes, which are physically felt. Students generally experience fatigue, thirst, or urinate frequently as the body releases toxins, but may also experience emotional and mental releases. This is common, especially after the first Aqualead class. This is why it is imperative that students rest after receiving an attunement. It is also preferable if people can wait longer, in order to have time to integrate the new knowledge and practise using the energy. Learning a healing modality requires a certain process, and each person has their own rhythm. The wait time, however, between the second level and Master level, is a minimum of four months. Before undertaking the Master level, students require more time and preparation, as well as more practice with the energy in order to be well acquainted with the energy and fully understand its meaning. The Aqualead Master level will be further discussed in another chapter.

The minimum age in order to receive an Aqualead attunement is five years old. The reason for this is that there now is an *Aqualead for Kids* Program in place, mainly for parents who are Aqualead Masters and desire teaching it to their children. The program is for children between the ages of five and 16 years.

Young children do not practise the full Aqualead session; they are attuned to the first symbols, and are made aware of the importance of connecting to water, nature and animals. The program for children is kept very simple at a young age. They can place their hands over a plant or animal, and transmit the energy healing for a short time. This introduction of Aqualead to children was gradual at the beginning, and not without some reserve and much precaution on my part. The energy was overwhelmingly strong at first, as it was new; however, as the adaptation phase progressed, the energy seemed a bit more manageable. I lowered the age limits; then, slowly, I allowed Aqualead to be taught to children, due to the high demand from Aqualead parents wanting to initiate their children to the energy.

As with the regular Aqualead Program, *Aqualead for Kids* has a definite guideline, set with age limits and contents for each level. The program for Kids has now been in place for a couple of years, with great success. Further practices and additions to the Aqualead Program will be discussed in subsequent chapters of this book.

vi. Communities worldwide

When it's time for a new energy to enter this world, it is interesting to see through whom the energy will manifest itself, and in what part of the world. I found it interesting, that being a Canadian living in the Gatineau region, just across the river from my place of birth, I did not channel Aqualead in the Ottawa Valley, in the comfort of my own back yard. Instead,

I ended up flying 6,000 miles away southward, to a remote country at the other end of the planet. For some reason, Aqualead needed to make its first entry into the world in Argentina: no place else. Of course I did not know the reason why I felt so drawn to Argentina when I left Canada in 2006. Nor was I expecting to go there on any special mission. What I do know is that the moment Aqualead appeared, I immediately understood the reason why I was there. I figure my guides who sent me this energy wanted it to make its arrival in that specific part of the world; there seems to be a lot more people learning and practising Aqualead in Argentina than anywhere else in the world. Perhaps people there are more ready and receptive to the new energy? Or maybe it has something to do with the proximity to Antarctica? Maybe my guides knew that the energy could spread far more quickly in the Americas and worldwide, through Argentina. I do know there is a deep connection between the energy of Aqualead and its birthplace, at the far end of South America.

After Aqualead became more established in Argentina, especially since spreading from within the country as of November 2009, it began reaching out to other countries, either through me or through other Masters. The two first Aqualead Masters from Mexico were taught in Puerto Iguazu, Misiones, Argentina in January 2010, when I visited Iguazu Falls on the Brazilian border. The first Aqualead Master from Uruguay was initiated in Capilla del Monte, Cordoba, by another Master and myself in March 2010. Next was Canada, where I initiated several Masters in the Ottawa region, when I returned home for a visit during the Christmas holidays in December 2010. Over a span of only a few years, Aqualead Masters appeared in Chile, Spain, Iceland, the United States, Norway, Sweden, Croatia, Brazil, Italy and Colombia. Meanwhile, Aqualead continued spreading massively throughout Argentina, in various provinces. In February 2013, I counted a total of 1,062 Aqualead Masters worldwide; 932 were in Argentina alone. In November 2012, there were 772 Aqualead Masters in Argentina. These figures include Aqualead Masters only; if all the practitioners were counted, the numbers could easily double. Due to the rapid growth of the modality in Argentina, I later established, with other Aqualead Masters, an *Aqualead Society* which oversees the quality of teaching nationwide.

It seems there was a necessity that Aqualead be here, and a new energy was anticipated in South America, which was readily receptive to it. Several of my students in Argentina commented to me the *urgent* feeling they had upon hearing about Aqualead. Many people commented that the Aqualead symbols seemed familiar to them when they first saw them. What was noticed from the beginning about Aqualead was the bonding experience it brings to all those who become involved with it. It seems the energy has a unifying effect on people, and tends to bring them together. It is common for Aqualead students to maintain friendships, organize gatherings and form a community. Aqualead practitioners and Masters tend to form large groups, like families. These families and groups are visible in social media, but also on a personal and individual level. As we continue working and advancing with this new energy, the connections between us will grow stronger as well. It seems the elevated awareness and the desire to protect and defend the Earth links us more to one another: to the Earth, to all life it harbours and to the elemental beings. Aqualead is here to remind us that we are not alone; we are all one, regardless of what part of the universe we come from.

PART I:

THE BIRTH OF AQUALEAD

CHAPTER I:

ORIGINS

i. Connecting to water

From the early stages of the development of life on the planet, water has been the beginning on Earth of all the living beings it supports. Any issues related to the environment are centred around a lack or a contamination of water. There has been a growing concern for the fate of the oceans and sources of drinkable water, as well as the future of life on Earth. Issues have being surfacing about what humanity puts in drinking water, as seen with chemicals added to the tap water. This is a time of rapid change and transformation in consciousness; and water is connecting us to this greater state of awareness. Within the past hundred years, some changes have been noticed in the Earth's climate, natural habitats and populations worldwide. Since the birth of the industrial era, there has been an increase in water, soil and air pollution, as well as deforestation, which brought certain species to the brink of extinction. The exploitation of fossil fuels and offshore drilling has put a stress on ecosystems and affected marine wildlife at an alarming rate.

With the appearance of all these signs of distress from destroyed natural habitats, animal and plant species, there has been a growing concern for our own future as a human race. We may ask ourselves: *For how long will the Earth hold out?* It seems that many efforts to improve the Earth's condition have been thwarted by a series of setbacks. However, despite these destructive patterns humanity has placed itself in, there is a Light growing, and this new Light has attracted some on a new path. This is a part of the shift that has been occurring since those past decades, as some changes began occurring unnoticed. Gradually, there has been an ever-growing desire in people everywhere to bring a change to the modern world's downward spiral. This is the awakening, as a new generation of people becoming healers and desiring to connect with nature and the Earth begin taking their stand, healing and teaching others.

Before the colonization of the Americas, the Native Peoples lived in harmony with nature and lived in a world of abundance, spirit and freedom. People took from the Earth only what they needed, and gave back in return, in the form of gratitude and acknowledgment. The Earth was considered a living, breathing being, and the Native People understood that the Earth could react and even retaliate if disrespected. Today, we see a renewed and increased interest in ancestral healing, and a greater general communion with the Earth. There is much more awareness and consciousness towards protecting and defending the planet. However, there is still a need for more growth and healing. A resistance is still coming from both the general population, as well as from those in power, who resist the change in order to serve their own interests.

In the light of this increased consciousness over the past 30 years, there has been an increase in the number of energy healers, learning different healing modalities, such as the practice of Reiki. These healing methods were labelled by many as esoteric or strange, as many of these practices were new and unknown at the time. The increase in the popularity of yoga, meditation and holistic therapies was greeted by some people with scepticism, and was still dismissed by the majority of people. Meanwhile, scientific journals and studies were much more trusted and recognized; ancient healing ways, such as herbal remedies and natural healing, were ignored and refuted. In this light, the use of crystals for healing or the practice of channelling messages from angels has been the object of disbelief and perceived as imagination.

Since then, there has been a gradual improvement as the spiritual healing communities have increased in strength and numbers. There are more yoga centres than before, and the practice of Tai Chi, Ayurveda and other holistic healing practices are making a comeback in the midst of the industrial modern age. A greater respect for alternative therapies has been noticed, as more and more people turn towards it, in order to find more holistic solutions to their health and personal issues. These problems can now be dealt with in a more holistic approach, encompassing the totality of a human being: *body, mind and spirit.* This higher state of spiritual awareness may seem to clash with the apparent escalation of violence occurring in different parts of the world; however, this violence is a resistance to the Light, as the Light continues to grow. And clearly, this transition phase we are crossing is not a smooth one.

In the light of this quiet green revolution occurring during the past couple of decades, the stage was being set for the arrival of Aqualead in our world. Now that we have passed through the cusp of the Aquarian Age since 2012, the transition is complete, yet the real transformation has only begun. We have noted this radical change in human consciousness, through the fact that in this new age of Light, *there are no secrets.* As the energy vibration in the world continues to increase, we see that lies, dissimulation and hypocrisies are increasingly more difficult to conceal. We have entered the age of truth, and these hidden realities will gradually come more into light, often in a frightening way. We are moving away from the age of illusions and fear. This process is a part of the purification that has begun occurring in the world in general. As with any healing process, the removal of dark, lower energies implies a certain amount of crisis, as we make room for higher vibrations of energy to enter, bringing more truth, genuine love and greater happiness.

The arrival of Aqualead in 2008 was timely in light of this need for more focus on environmental issues, such as habitat destruction and animal abuse. It seems that issues of deforestation, water and air contamination and general violence were still ongoing and left unresolved. There was also seemingly a need for a new tool that would enable one to work in a deeper, more focused way on the Earth and the planet itself. With the widespread use, practice and knowledge of Reiki worldwide, it seems that the change was still insufficient and incomplete. There also seemed to be a vast range of knowledge about angels and Ascended Masters, however, little knowledge or awareness about nature beings or *elemental beings*. I felt there was something missing in my range of healing practice, even though I didn't know what it was until later on.

What lead us even closer to the coming of Aqualead was the work of Japanese scientist Masaru Emoto and his observation of water crystals. His pictures of water crystals showed how water responded to our thoughts, words and emotions, and changed accordingly. It was then clear to everyone that water is intelligent and has the ability to react to its surroundings. The topic of water took a strong importance in everyone's minds, and this awareness put ourselves and life on Earth in their proper perspective: first of all, we are all one. We are all connected, since we are made of the same element, *regardless of species*. Second, when we hurt others, we only hurt ourselves. Any form of violence and victimization towards others is counter-productive, and will only result in backfiring, causing suffering to the perpetrator. Seeing how this fundamental, life-supporting element can react, and carries its own consciousness, revealed to us the necessity to re-examine how we treat others and how we treat ourselves. This revelation and new understanding of water resulted in greater wisdom, more respect and a new insight about how we treat this planet.

In the midst of all this, Aqualead made its appearance in the most unexpected and unusual way. Looking back, I am now convinced that my decision to leave for Argentina in 2006 from the comfort of my home in Canada was not mere coincidence. Unannounced and unknown, this new energy made its way and found me there, in order to be translated into new knowledge. I did not yet know what this was I was scribbling on a torn piece of paper that evening, while at work in downtown Buenos Aires. Yet it somehow made complete sense; and the very first message I received as I drew the first symbol was that this was supposed to *heal water.*

ii. Background

Before leaving Canada for South America, I had already felt a strong desire to change my life. However, I did not have the resources, knowledge or exposure to receive the necessary guidance to achieve this. What followed were a series of steps I was guided to take in order to ultimately prepare for this exile to Argentina. The year 2003 proved to be a turning point for me, as I began developing an interest in spirituality, meditation and reading tarot cards. I started reading various books on the subject, and realized I had unused abilities that needed nurturing. I also recognized that there were certain parts of my life that I felt needed healing, in order to be able to move on. As I continued educating myself and discovering the world of holistic healing, meditation, yoga and Runes, I encountered another turning point in my life, which was when I took my first Reiki class in Ottawa. Having no clue what this was, or why I felt so compelled to do this, I walked into my Reiki Master's small classroom, apprehensive, nervous and not knowing what would happen next. I just felt an invisible force carrying me every step of the way, and I never hesitated or questioned it. After completing my first level of Reiki, I started my Kundalini yoga teacher training in a yoga school in Ottawa, in January 2005. My next turning point appeared to me during the first weekend of this intensive yoga training; after doing exercises in breathing, chanting mantras and meditations, I received a message the following morning at home to change my diet to become vegetarian. This message clearly came through telling me to *stop eating beef and pork*, as clear as I could understand someone speaking to me, in thought. I immediately felt compelled to do so without any hesitation; somehow this abrupt change of diet felt natural and beneficial to me, and I have remained vegetarian and later vegan ever since.

It seems I simply followed one transition after another, growing on the personal and spiritual level, and I felt after each change and turn, that I should never look back. As of June 2005, I continued my Reiki levels and became a Reiki Master later in the same year, and began learning other healing modalities, and discovering healing with angels. With the series of attunements I had received from other modalities that I had learned, such as an angelic healing technique, healing with an Ascended Master and later a more advanced style of Reiki, my intuition began to sharpen and I started connecting to angels, spirit guides and other ascended Masters. I realized I was able to communicate with the spirit world with relative ease, as I could *hear (clairaudiently)* messages from the *other side*. This led me to the new skill of channelling, which consists of writing down messages from spiritual and angelic beings. The beings I was channelling from were my own spirit guides and guardian angels, and I also found myself at times communicating with people who had passed on, effortlessly. I began teaching psychic development classes and hosting small psychic gatherings with friends and students at my home. This is how I eventually wrote and published my first book, *The Psychic's Guide, Volume One* in May 2005, based on my psychic development classes. Another burst of creativity led me to the release of my first set of oracle cards entitled *Women of the Earth*, published in Ottawa in 2006.

As I grew and changed, I realized just how much I had become different from the people I had known, and how far I had gone in my personal journey of transformation. To many people around me, I began appearing strange, being all at once a vegan, an energy healer and practising a strange and ancient style of yoga. I began distancing myself from certain areas of my life, such as work, and in early 2006, I challenged the boundaries of my personal safety by quitting my job with the City of Ottawa, where I was working as a paramedic. At this point I had moved back to my mother's home on the Québec shore of the Ottawa River, and had already planned a change in career which entailed travel and languages. I enjoyed the idea of leaving the country, and working abroad while travelling. Teaching English abroad seemed like the perfect venture for me. I just felt I needed a change in my life, and was aiming at a new career as an English as a Second Language teacher.

After much time and research, I finally took a short English as a Second Language teacher course. This new background, series of events and changes in my life led to my departure from Ottawa, Canada, in September 2006 for Buenos Aires. I had never set foot in South America before, and I knew only some basic knowledge of Spanish through previous visits to Cuba. I was hurling myself into the great unknown, but somehow I trusted that I had to go to Argentina and that something important awaited me there. However, for the time being, I was going on a journey of discovery, hoping to teach some English and gain experience while there. Upon my arrival in Buenos Aires, I stayed in a small hostel in the city, and began my journey from there. I met new friends, other yoga teachers and began practising at a yoga centre, through a teacher I met there. I ended up moving to a house in Argentina with an Argentine family, in the barrio of *Caballito.* I lived there for one and a half years. I found living with Argentines most helpful during my first months in Buenos Aires, where I was able to pick up some language and learn to speak *Castellano.* I then became familiar with local football teams, such as *Boca Juniors.* I also discovered *mate* (pronounced ma-tay), the Argentine tea which is drunk in a gourd, and drawn up with a small pipe *(bombilla),* in a similar fashion to a straw. I slowly started knowing the city better, improved my Spanish and understood the Argentine accent in conversation. I began teaching Kundalini yoga in a yoga centre in a suburb of Buenos Aires called *Martinez,* and began teaching Reiki around the same time. I adapted and translated my materials to Spanish, in order to accommodate my new Argentine friends and students. My adaptation into Argentine society and way of life was, despite the early culture shock upon my arrival, smooth and flowed naturally.

It was throughout my stay at the house in Caballito that I met and connected with new Argentine friends and colleagues who would later become my students and play a prominent role in the development of Aqualead. My circle of friends in Argentina included a tourist from Iceland who stayed in Buenos Aires in order to practise tango. She had contacted me in order to take classes with me. She made three trips to Buenos Aires; I taught her during each of her visits and we remained friends afterwards. I continued teaching Reiki and later initiated some new Reiki Masters. I worked and frequently went for walks in downtown Buenos Aires in Plaza de Mayo, near the *Pink House* (parliament). I taught business English for a year at a language institute, and later landed a job in a call centre in technical support, in the downtown core of Buenos Aires. This secured me a work visa and allowed me to stay in the country with residential status. In December 2007, I made my first visit to Canada in order to spend time with family during the holidays. I promptly returned to Argentina after the New Year. In June 2008, I moved to an apartment in the barrio of *Almagro*, Buenos Aires. It was at this apartment that a series of strange and peculiar events began occurring that would later change my life forever.

iii. The channelling process

While living in Argentina, I felt deeply concerned about the state of the environment, and the astounding amount of air and water pollution that surrounded me. I already felt the urge to do healing work on the Earth, and often sent energy healing to the planet, the environment surrounding me and to the oceans. I felt the Earth needed to be cleansed of all this contamination, which was placed into the water by cities everywhere. I used all the tools that I had received from my Reiki training, and thought this was as much as I could do at the environmental level. I continued reading books on the subject of energy healing, and had acquired a book about water and consciousness, written by Japanese scientist Masaru Emoto. I was fascinated by the photographs of the water crystals, and how our thoughts and feelings could change them. However, I still did not know how to integrate and incorporate this information into my healing work, and I had never before heard of an energy specifically focused on healing water.

One Saturday evening, I was at work at the call centre sitting in my cubicle waiting for a next call. It was a very quiet evening and I was reading the book on water. It was around seven o'clock. I finished the final chapter in the book, and put it down. After a few moments, a vision came to my mind, and it appeared to me as an image of a drop of water. The image seemed persistent and strong in my mind's eye, and I felt the urge to copy the image on a piece of paper. I tore a piece of paper next to me, and with a pen I drew the picture. It seemed to be a symbol, because as I drew it, more details of the picture appeared while I was tracing it. More lines appeared, seeming like waves; however, the image was specific and seemed to represent something. I knew this was not only an art project. At that point, I received a clear message that this symbol was to heal water. That's when I realized and received confirmation that this was an energy healing symbol, and not a mere scribble landing by chance. I was thrilled that something appeared to me in relation to water, as a means to heal it. I did not receive too much detail about the symbol afterwards. I thought this channelling process was over, and was contemplating this new finding with wonder.

But as soon as the first image was completed, a second symbol appeared and as I drew it, it seemed even more complicated than the first, because I was drawing hooks around it. The next symbol appeared like ocean waves, and the fourth, another drop of water with different features. I had never seen such symbols before; however, I felt they were important. I felt a presence throughout this process; but I did not pay too much attention as to who was present, because I was so absorbed and intrigued by what was happening. However, after the four symbols were physically drawn on paper, my informant did not allow me to rest.

More information came through, this time in the form of words. The knowledge of names for these symbols somehow appeared in my mind, and I did not pause to question this information, or where it came from. I just followed it. What followed felt like a guessing game, perhaps in the form of riddles, and my informant would tell me whether I was correct or not. I had to make out the names of the symbols, one letter at a time, because they were so strange, until the correct name was spelled out. There seemed to be an understanding between me and my visitor (I felt more than one presence at this point). In order to write the name, I first had to ask how many letters there were in the name. For example, the name for the first symbol I channelled had four letters, and my informant would confirm to me whether this was correct. I would then ask whether the first letter was a vowel or a consonant. The first letter was a consonant. I would then go through all the consonants in the alphabet until the correct sound or pronunciation was matched. This is how I knew that the first letter of the first symbol was *Z*. I would then get positive confirmation of this in order to make sure I was right. The second letter was an *A*, and so forth, until the full name of the symbol was revealed. I carefully wrote down these names on the torn piece of paper next to the appropriate symbol, and in my notepad. This process took only a few minutes for each symbol. Each of the four symbols had their own name.

I soon realized that this was not only a group of separate symbols; this was a healing modality, a fully functional system, I concluded, as more information was given to me. The symbols were quickly divided into three levels: the first level had one symbol, the second level had another and the third level had the two remaining symbols. I then learned the function or purpose of each symbol. Except for only one, the symbols were focused on facets of healing water in living beings and on the rest of the planet. What I felt was a combination of surprise, amazement and overall shock. All of this happened as I sat quietly in my chair. Not once did I have a moment of doubt, suspicion or apprehension. And despite the fact that this information was completely unknown, as well as the source of this information, I never had a single inkling of fear or worry.

My informants provided me with more information. At this stage, I felt like a student taking notes from invisible teachers who dictated to me. I was given a related colour for three of the symbols, and each was a shade of blue; then a different crystal was associated with each of the same three symbols. At this point I began feeling a deep gratitude towards my informants for providing me or sending me all this information. When I look back, I wonder if my informants were present with me in the room, or if they were sending me this information telepathically at a distance. Regardless, the information I received was clear, precise and simply made sense to me. Also, what was peculiar was the presence I felt of an angel, whose name I heard was *Ariel.* There was no name yet for this new modality to be used for healing water; I simply called it *water energy healing*, for the sake of attributing the modality a name. This was the bulk of the initial channelling process. It was clearly unplanned, unintended and mostly unexpected. I was fully awake, in a normal state. I was fully aware and conscious of my surroundings throughout the entire exchange of information.

After the end of my shift at work, I went straight home with this information in my bag and once there, I immediately began typing all this information as a document in my laptop. I automatically created three documents, one for each level to be taught. It was only the following day that the actual name of the modality was received. It was during the afternoon, and I was walking on the street in Buenos Aires near where I lived, after doing some small groceries. The name sounded like something *aquatic* and had the *aqua* component to it. After trial and error, and checking with my new masters and with angel Ariel, who was still present at the time, we finally agreed upon the correct name: *AQUALEAD*. As soon I arrived home, I wrote this name down and saved it.

iv. About angel Ariel

I have always loved angels, believed in angels and have had a deep respect and reverence for these loving beings who act as protective healers and messengers in our world. Even though I felt the presence of an angel throughout this channelling process, I clearly felt there were other beings present or involved in this process. I do know that this information did not come from angel Ariel alone, as I initially believed. These other beings who sent me the information were mostly male, however, there was a female; these distant masters were mainly a group of four or five. These people were clearly not angels, or human; they lived in a distant world and possessed immense powers. I now fully understand and realize that this angel was present during this process to assist in the actual reception of this new information, a bit like a mediator or a translator. Angels are something familiar and common in this world. The knowledge and understanding of angels is widespread, either through different religious traditions, different spiritual healing practices, or as an icon of peace on Earth during Christmas season, celebrated worldwide. Perhaps this angel's presence was necessary at this time as a messenger, as I could not know or fully understand the actual origins of this healing energy. The angel provided me with a familiar reference, as I was treading into completely unknown and unchartered territory.

What I noticed also was the feeling of a very high and pure vibration of energy. As I channelled this information on paper in written form, I had a sense of a very cleansing energy, as if the coolest and purest water had entered my body and my soul. I felt that this energy had a very cleansing effect on the human body, mind and spirit. In the light of all the environmental pollution, which is inevitably linked to water contamination, I felt that the arrival of this energy was timely and most needed. This truly felt to me as though a birthing process was taking place, however, I never realized until later the magnitude of what I was doing. I do feel the angel's presence was important during this channelling process, to remove any doubts or fears, and perhaps protect the space from any potential negative interference, as I put down this information on paper with pen.

I must admit that my knowledge of angels is generally limited. There are many healers and different clairvoyants everywhere who specialize in this field of energy work, and can perform healing and counselling work with different angels and archangels. Others give clairvoyant readings by connecting with angelic beings and using angel oracle cards, while others channel different books and messages from angels. I never did much of the sort. I had received in the past some training in angelic healing, but my knowledge of the whole angelic hierarchy remained limited. I know that angel Ariel is also correlated to a certain angelic technique I had learned; but I do know that in this case, there was no connexion whatsoever between this healing method and what I had just channelled. I had a sense also that angel Ariel is not an archangel (even though the pronunciation of the name is reminiscent of archangel *Uriel*). I had a feeling that angel Ariel was perhaps a seraph angel, of a higher ranking order than the archangels. She appeared to me as very tall and luminescent.

Shortly after the initial stages of the channelling phase, angel Ariel gave this blessing that I wrote down concerning Aqualead and its healing purpose on the planet. Again, I am by no means an angel specialist or a usual channeller of angelic information, but this blessing was maintained and shared among all practitioners in the Aqualead community. I also do feel this message is important, relevant and nice to share with others, for its simplicity and supportiveness:

Blessing from Angel Ariel:

"The human body is composed mostly of water. Likewise, most of planet Earth's surface is covered with water. Water in your world is a precious gift of life. In order to heal the Earth and all its inhabitants, all its water must be purified and healed, in order to heal all the life forms it sustains. Healing and cleansing all the water on planet Earth, including the water inside your physical bodies, means healing the body, mind and emotions in order to bring a new level of clarity and balance. This is a crucial time for your world to heal itself and for the planet to restore its natural state, and the angels are there to assist humanity throughout these important changes. Healing and cleansing the water inside your bodies will bring on a new healing vibration to the Earth. This means healing the oceans that surround you, as well as the ocean within. The human consciousness is a vast ocean, let alone the physical body. Animals, plants, trees are also the embodiment of this divine gift of life. Like all living creatures, the Earth itself needs its water

cleansed, purified and rejuvenated in order to create a heavenly new world, free of harmful toxins.

This is why we share this new energy with you, dear ones, so we can work together and manifest a new healing life force within all living beings, on planet Earth. This healing vibration is no different from the energy of pure love and gratitude offered to all the water on this planet, found within all its creatures, its vegetation and within you."

- September 2nd, 2008

This blessing from the angels carries a message of love for the planet and a desire to help rebalance the Earth and all the life it supports. This also indicated to me the desire of beings from outside this world to assist the Earth and humanity in its evolution. Despite the close connection from working with this angel throughout the beginnings of Aqualead, this energy did not originate from the angels. It has a very high angelic vibration, however, the origin or the source of Aqualead was revealed to me only at a later time, as I continued working with this energy and channelling more information. Also, despite the religious connotations angels generally tend to carry, Aqualead is not a religion and it is not limited to Christianity.

v. The galaxy next door

I knew from the beginning of the entire process that Aqualead was an energy that was *not from here.* Much more than just a universal energy, this was an angelic energy, or related to the angelic realm; I simply understood and acknowledged that. This was partially true. After some years of experience working with other different healing energies such as Reiki, I already had the concept in my mind of what a universal energy would be. To me, Aqualead constituted a universal energy as it came from beyond this world, and surely beyond this part of the universe. After this initial phase of channelling, I later realized, or rather was later signalled by my guides, that Aqualead is actually an energy coming from *another planet.* It was only in 2010 that I would become informed that Aqualead not only comes from another part of the universe but from a specific location called the *Andromeda galaxy.* When my guides informed me of this, I received the message suddenly while alone in my apartment. The message came loud and clear.

I had never before heard of energies coming from this specific place, nor did I have any previous information about Andromeda. After a brief check online, I saw that Andromeda is the nearest spiralling galaxy to our own, which is called the *Milky Way.* Upon receiving this information about the origins of Aqualead, I felt rather uneasy. That is not to say that I am intimidated by the idea of the existence of life on other planets. And the idea of the existence of extraterrestrial beings did not concern me either. It was rather from a standpoint of how to tell and explain this information to others, when first of all I am not an astronomer; second, there is no scientific or factual proof that there are inhabited worlds with intelligent life *out there*. The very idea of telling the general population that I had channelled a new healing energy and that it came from the Andromeda galaxy intimidated me. I could already imagine the scepticism and ridicule that would follow.

Despite my fear of how people would react, I felt upon receiving this bit of information a nudge inside me, like a confirmation that this could be real. It just felt right, like a sense of inner trust, and the thought of Aqualead energy being from Andromeda no longer worried me. Still, I kept this information to myself until later on; however, my concerns proved to be unfounded as I gradually told my students and the information was welcomed. The knowledge of Aqualead being an *extraterrestrial energy* grew stronger in me, as I felt this energy and worked with it more over the years. Something I had noticed about this energy was its vibrant presence and the unusual feeling it gave off. This energy felt very intense to me, like something very ancient coming from afar. This only confirmed to me even more that Aqualead was actually not from this galaxy, and could in fact be *Andromedan*. As I discovered the link between the energy and this distant galaxy, I was also learning about what such an energy could change within this world.

This knowledge had allowed me to trace more of the possible history and background of this new energy before I made first contact with it through angel Ariel. It also gave me more insight as to where this energy came from, what its origins were, and who were these beings that I call *my masters.* Aqualead's presence in my life changed many things in me on the physical, mental and emotional levels. But more than that, this energy also changed my view of the universe, this planet we live on, and my relationship with nature and the environment. Discovering the true origins of Aqualead also allowed me to ascertain that this world is receiving *outside help* from an intelligent source, with the purpose of healing, balancing and hopefully helping to break humanity's destructive patterns here on Earth. Without this help from the outside, Aqualead would otherwise not have arrived here. I am sure of that; and I am certain that the arrival of this energy in our world was not at random, nor was it an accident or coincidence of any kind.

CHAPTER II:

STEPPING OUT

i. Writing the first manuals

When I began entering the initial information about Aqualead, which was basically the four symbols and the name *Aqualead*, I typed out the information in my laptop in the form of three documents, which ended up serving as templates for the eventual first Aqualead manuals. There was a question in my mind as to whether there should be three or four levels in the Aqualead healing system, but the answer soon came to me that there should be three levels only. The main reason was to maintain the simplicity of the modality, with a simple yet accessible structure, while focusing instead on the power of the energy itself. The writing began as soon as I came home from work that very same evening I received the first information. It seemed normal and natural to me, perhaps I felt guided to do so, to create right away the three first manuals and several other documents as I was carefully saving this information. It was clear to me from the beginning that this energy modality would not be kept secret for long, but I visibly needed time to develop and elaborate certain aspects of it. The actual procedure as to how to give an Aqualead healing session was already established while I was still at work, which was rather simple. However, the other thing that was missing was the attunement process, in order to teach this and eventually enable others to practise it.

If a healing modality is to be functional, it must not only be taught to others in order to spread; it must also be able to perpetuate itself indefinitely, and create a lineage of Masters, or those empowered to teach it. What ensures that a modality can survive is when teachers can initiate or train other teachers. It seems my new Masters or guides already read my mind about my many questions and concerns about this. From the beginning, there was already a Master level and an attunement symbol established in the healing system, hence my train of questioning. They provided me with the steps to the attunement process soon after, while I was in my small room, in the apartment where I was living on Medrano Street. The process was simple, and more simplified than other attunement processes I'd learned before, through other healing modalities. This initial information was saved, and added to the document for the third level. At that point, with a general procedure for an Aqualead healing session, and a procedure for an Aqualead Master to give attunements at each level, I felt that I finally had a fully functioning healing modality. But still, more things were yet to happen.

Within days after August 30th, I began receiving the actual energy itself. Now that the initial information about the energy and the Aqualead modality was written, it was time for me to experience the energy first-hand. I found this difficult at the beginning, because I was the very first person in this world to make physical contact with this strange new energy. Also, I had no one to share these experiences with, because I could not tell friends and acquaintances about this energy I had just received. The energy came to me directly from the *source*, as opposed to through the hands of a human master; this, I believe, made the experience altogether different for me. This also allowed me to become acquainted with the energy in a very personal and intimate way. I received the energy of Aqualead over a span of three or four days, in three different waves, which I associate with each level of Aqualead. I found this process overall unpleasant, if not at some point physically painful, but it was necessary before I could even begin using and practising this energy. What I hadn't realized either was how much the arrival of this powerful new energy would wreak havoc inside a home or building.

The first wave of energy was relatively smooth. I felt the cleansing release in my body; it felt strong and I soon realized from this first experience that this was not anything like other healing energies I was accustomed to. This clearly *was not Reiki.* The energy felt to me as cooling, refreshing, clean and gave me the sensation of fresh spring water. It felt very cleansing. What also struck me was the intensity of this energy, very vibrant, as if it wanted to pounce on anything that had water in it. From the beginning I have described Aqualead as being a very dynamic, fast acting energy that may at times work aggressively in order to release any pollutants, contaminants or negative energy. As much as Reiki has more of a pacifying, harmonizing and gentle feel to it, Aqualead felt more, by comparison, like the tiger ready to leap forward, or a shark ready to strike at the speed of lightning. I felt this energy could do a lot in a world like ours, on such a damaged, polluted and distressed planet.

I expected the second wave of energy to be like the first. It would be the equivalent of sampling a new wine in a restaurant, taking the time to smell and feel in every detail its aroma and texture. This is not what happened. After my guides told me I was to receive the second wave of Aqualead energy, I went to bed that evening, and that's when the pain started. I was not yet asleep, when I suddenly felt a sharp, stabbing pain in my right flank. The pain was so intense, I thought my right kidney or liver was about to explode; I couldn't move or breathe. After lying immobilized in bed for what seemed like an eternity, I felt a presence practically forcing me to get up and go to the bathroom. I thought this was impossible. Still, I managed to get up with this excruciating flank pain, and slowly walked bent forward to the bathroom, and went back to my room. I wanted to lie down again, but my guide present with me would not allow me. I was instructed to walk around. Against my will, I began doing that; I walked in circles in my small room, wondering whether I would survive the night. I am not sure whether this being was present with me in the room, or someone talking to me from far away. However, I knew by then that I no longer felt angel Ariel's presence or involvement with the development of Aqualead. This pain lasted for about another hour and a half. After some time, I began coughing. It started as a dry cough, but then became more productive, and I began coughing out a strange *sputum*. And I started spitting it out; it appeared like small, yellow chunks, almost like pieces of butter. I continued coughing for a while like this; then eventually the coughing stopped. I was later able to go back to bed and get some sleep for the rest of the night.

As much as I trusted my guides and masters at this point, I was apprehensive and almost fearful of receiving the third of these series of energies. My experience with the second direct attunement I had received was quite painful; one hour had felt like three. I understood that the strange sputum I was coughing out and the entire pain I felt was a release in my body from the new energy. I had enough experience in the world of energy healing to understand that often a healing crisis could be unpleasant, uncomfortable and even upsetting. But I had never in my life experienced a pain such as this one before. However, I knew I had already gone too far to turn back; and stopping this process was not an option. After a couple of days, I received the third wave of energy, which actually felt to me as though a blessing had come upon me. The experience was far less traumatic, and it seemed I had passed the worst of it. Again it felt stronger than the second, minus the pain and the intense physical releasing. It was rather a more emotional releasing that I felt, and I remember that it began raining moments after the third phase of the energy had reached me. I also remember one my new guides telling me that I had now become an Aqualead Master, and that I was now able to give attunements.

At this point I began noticing the effect this new energy had on machines, electronic appliances, especially relating to water. It shouldn't be surprising, when you consider that the third level of Aqualead enables one to move water. Suddenly, the power of nature which moves water is finding itself contained inside a pipe within the walls of a building. In the apartment where I lived, we began experiencing a series of plumbing issues after the final wave of the energy had passed. Over the span of the few months I was living there, the toilet would not work, and the shower was smashed down by plumbers in order to find a faulty water pipe. The washing machine wouldn't work, and then later we had no water at all. And finally, water began seeping through one of the walls just outside of my room, and the entire living room floor of the apartment was covered with two inches of water. I remember this flooding occurred twice in the apartment. However, there was never a drop of water in my bedroom, which I found interesting. I also remember going to a print shop nearby to photocopy the very first images of the Aqualead symbols to be added to manuals, and the photocopy machine breaking down. This initial reaction to the new energy soon passed, however, and things went back to normal.

ii. With the help of friends

It was now the month of September of 2008, and I was still the only person to know about Aqualead. I knew I still needed time to get accustomed to this energy, to get to know it and to practise it. I had started giving myself self-healing treatments, and the energy did feel to me as genuine, real and unique. However, being alone with this made it difficult for me to determine whether I was truly accurate, or if this was all just my imagination. Perhaps, after all of this, what I discovered was simply a variation of an energy I already had previously. I knew that at some point I would have to show my findings to other reliable and experienced healers, and get their feedback. It was only towards the beginning of October that I felt it was time to send an email to a small group of friends and healers that I knew; all of them had been my students at some point, however, some were very experienced and knowledgeable. I emailed a group of six people, and for the first time I told them about this new energy I had received called Aqualead. I offered to meet with them and try out a session to see how they felt about it.

This being an unknown energy, I expected apprehension, fear, worry or suspicion from my friends. However, the response from all of them was immediately positive. One friend of mine, who was already an experienced healer using various techniques, was enthusiastic and eager to try it. I decided to meet with my friend Andrés first, and get his opinion about it. Andrés is a young Reiki Master in Buenos Aires and had taken an interest in my psychic development work; this is how he had previously contacted me for classes, and we later became friends. He is also an avid meditator and is open to other energy healing modalities, including the use of gongs and other Tibetan musical instruments. His help turned out to be a crucial turning point in the development of Aqualead. After the channelling work was done, I could not go further without the assistance of others, who would receive the energy and give me their feedback, and who would eventually learn it, and teach it to others. There is no such thing as a teacher without a student. Early in October, I went to Andrés' apartment in downtown Buenos Aires; after a brief discussion and explaining to him about this new energy and how it came to me, he was ready and eager to try it. He lay there on the floor and I began giving him the first Aqualead session. At the end of the session, he gave an overall positive feedback about the energy, and how he felt it. Based on his feedback, this definitely was not Reiki or any other existing healing energy. This for me was important, as I could not confirm this alone. I asked him if he wanted to learn it and try out the first level; however, I warned him that this energy was completely new, and no one had ever received an Aqualead attunement before. Andrés was not fazed; we set a date to meet in the healing office where he was practising and the first Aqualead class was already set.

From then on I was amazed at the amount of faith and trust my friends in Argentina demonstrated about Aqualead. From the beginning, no one had ever expressed any doubt or fear about receiving this energy; on the contrary. It seemed right, and flowed perfectly well. I also noticed how Aqualead's entry into this world would be no less than a slow adaptation to a higher vibration. I also understood that this new energy would pose a challenge to all of us, regardless if a person who encountered Aqualead was already an experienced energy healer or a rank beginner. The message of Aqualead was that abundance comes from faith and trust in the universe and the elements that surround us; and that what we send out will come back to us tenfold. The emphasis on this new energy was about healing the Earth from the beginning, and this is something that my guides made clear with me from the beginning. That was not going to be a simple energy healing modality; Aqualead went beyond that, as a way of life and a new way of dealing with environmental issues that would otherwise have left us feeling helpless. Aqualead was here to instigate profound changes in this world, not only at the environmental level, but at the personal and human level, as a platform to personal growth.

iii. Early experiences

Soon after my initial experience with Andrés, I started off to a small suburb outside of the city limits of Buenos Aires, in *zona Norte*. There, I met three friends and healers at a friend's house, who were students of mine. One by one, I gave them an Aqualead session; they were baffled. One of the ladies commented, after finishing the session, that she had a vision of an angel pouring water over her from a vase from above, throughout the session. Someone else commented, after her turn, that she felt an intense heat in my hands, even though my hands were not placed directly on her. What they had experienced was definitely not Reiki, which we were all accustomed to using. The feedback and excitement were unanimous about this new healing energy, and they had given me the additional confidence and confirmation I needed. They were all eager to start learning Aqualead. Later in the month came the first Aqualead classes ever taught. This was only the first of a series of important breakthroughs, as Aqualead continued to grow and develop. It seemed as though the energy simply lead the way, and all I had to do was to follow its lead. Visibly this energy appeared intelligent to me, with a higher consciousness, and knew exactly where and how it had to proceed. I simply trusted Aqualead, and let it decide for itself what was to come next.

I met with Andrés again, at the little studio he was sharing with other healing practitioners in the city, for our Aqualead class. I arrived in the bright little apartment and he greeted me as I came out of the elevator. Needless to say, we both knew this was purely experimental, and at this point it was a trial, trying out a new energy and finally *testing* the attunement. In the early stages of Aqualead, there wasn't much to teach at the first level. There was only one symbol, where to place the hands in a session, distant healing and give the attunement. I gave him the attunement; the energy felt powerful in my hands, however manageable. There was no obvious reaction in my student either. His comments on the attunement were overall positive, and it seemed like a normal attunement, uneventful, without any major discomfort. I was relieved. And now came the real test: have the student practise the session on me. I had never received an Aqualead session from anyone yet, since I was the only person capable of giving it. He placed his hands above me and I saw a cool stream of clear water and waterfalls. The energy was powerful, intense, and at the same time I could feel a strong heat under the practitioner's hands; this was not the familiar Reiki anymore as we had clearly moved beyond. I was amazed and fascinated by this, and I knew right away that this energy was not anything known in this world. The trial was a success.

Soon after, I taught the first level of Aqualead to my small group of students at my friend's house. They all received the attunement, and began practising Aqualead on one another as well as on me. We all knew this new energy was real, and I knew this was going to move forward. I next began teaching the second level of Aqualead to my student and to the others in *zona Norte*. That's when we started focusing more on the environmental level with the symbol, and sending it at a distance. I also heard feedback from students experiencing releasing symptoms after receiving the attunement, such as flu-like symptoms. However the cleansing crisis occurred, it was never like that painful experience I had had at the apartment where I lived. More people began practising the self-healing session, and I was already busy sending Aqualead energy at a distance, as I continued preparing for classes and noting observations on the energy itself.

It is interesting to note that usually when something new appears, such as a new healing energy, one would normally take the time (months or years) to carefully develop the modality before first trying it with others. However, this did not occur with Aqualead. Rather, the energy seemed to want to make contact with people right away, and would not allow me to keep it behind closed doors, in order to get to know it more. The trials and experimenting were meant to be shared among others. Perhaps, also, I felt the energy simply wanted to make its way outward as soon as possible to healers who could begin sending the energy to rivers and oceans, and everywhere else. I can't help but think that this was related to the energy's personality, which was expressive, colourful and outgoing. It seems Aqualead simply wanted to act through human beings as soon as possible in order to initiate its work, and my students in Argentina responded to that feeling of urgency, by getting this energy out and putting it to use right away. We soon began sending energy to the river nearby, called *Rio de la Plata*, and to the oceans and lakes in and around Argentina. All rivers in Argentina are polluted, however, it was interesting to note that at times I could feel a dark energy releasing from the water when sending Aqualead. Sometimes this energy could be seen intuitively, appearing as a black cloud or smoke lifting from it. Some friends and I occasionally went to the river and physically sat near the water, in order to perform the healing work with Aqualead.

On October 26th, 2008, I met with my student Andrés again for the third time, this time for the Aqualead Master level class. Again, this was a first; this first Aqualead Master class was very simple, since there were at the time only two symbols to teach. After giving him the attunement, I opened my eyes, and I felt as though the world had just changed. He practised the attunement on me. This was my very first time receiving an Aqualead attunement, after practising and teaching it for some time. It felt interesting, as I could feel the vibrant energy working at the back of my head; however, I felt without a doubt that I was receiving an attunement. This day marked another breakthrough; then, we brainstormed some ideas as to what could be useful and incorporated into the Aqualead levels. I already had some ideas, and Andrés' input proved helpful, especially for the Master level.

On November 2nd, I taught another Aqualead Master class at my friend's house. The ladies practised the attunement there, and from then on, I just knew that Aqualead would travel and circulate on its own, from one Aqualead Master to other new Masters, and so forth. The Aqualead modality proved to be valid, safe and fully functional in the world. One thing that appealed to me about Aqualead is the fact that it remained free of charge. I also realized that Aqualead being free of charge would require some adaptation from certain people on the personal, social and mental levels. The fact that Aqualead was free was established from the beginning, by my new masters. There were two reasons for this: first of all, because the energy's purpose was to heal the Earth. Due to its very high vibration of energy and elemental origins, this energy was not to become a business or the object of a commercial endeavour. The Aqualead sessions and classes remain free of charge, but voluntary donations are accepted. This made Aqualead into a non-profit organization, which seemed perfect given the context of its origins and purpose. Healing the Earth and water in this world was something that is priceless, especially with this new energy that was so generously sent to us to heal it. The second reason why Aqualead was free from the start is because my guides asked that it remained so.

This new energy's presence posed a challenge, not only to all healers but to all of us as human beings. This challenge consisted of using this energy, practising it and teaching it for free, solely for the welfare of the Earth and the restoration of nature, while remaining detached from any expectation of a financial gain. However, the return from teaching Aqualead classes for free was, I found, far greater than being handed money charged as a fee. Charging money for Aqualead simply did not make sense and it became obvious to some of us that this energy did not resonate with the common concepts of *business* and *money*. This energy was elemental and unique, and was not to be treated like other healing systems. This modality was centred around an act of love, generosity and gratitude towards the Earth. Being free of charge also made the modality widely accessible and available to everyone, without any discrimination.

In December 2008, I flew back to Canada for my second visit to family and friends. It was a short visit, but many things were achieved over a short period of time. This is when I taught the first level of Aqualead to a student in Ottawa. I also gave an attunement to a student at home on the Québec side. It was during this visit back home, that I first made a definitive connection with elemental beings. They appeared to me directly in my mother's house, and I began noticing them, tall and slender, some with brown, black or platinum blonde hair; I knew they were Elves. It seemed that they appeared to me because they knew I would be able to see them and communicate with them. It was not frightened at all; they communicated to me telepathically, and clearly understood my thoughts. It seems to me that during those moments, my perception of things had changed. It was also apparent that my notion of time had changed, and that I had somehow shifted into a parallel dimension. The whole encounter seemed to me a bit surreal, and I also could feel my guides and masters speaking to me more clearly, with a firm and protective guidance surrounding me. With this new sudden change in my life, I left my mother's house in Gatineau, Québec, and returned back to Buenos Aires.

iv. On the road

Back in Buenos Aires, I slowly continued teaching Aqualead and initiating more Masters. I noticed that

I was getting fewer Aqualead students in the capital city of Buenos Aires. The energy seemed to often want to go outside of city limits, to the quieter and greener neighbourhoods of *zona Norte*, namely in *Martinez*, where I met and taught my friends Lupe and Marian. I was connected to them through a lady with whom I was teaching English in downtown Buenos Aires. I commuted to this area on numerous occasions, and I eventually had many students coming to me from that area outside of Buenos Aires. I observed that the energy had a very bonding effect among people, and I found myself being connected from one person to the next, as I taught; one student had a friend whom they knew would be interested in Aqualead, and so forth. Starting in 2009, I began travelling more. Marian, one of my new Aqualead students who lived in Martinez, had a long-time friend living in the south of Argentina, in Bariloche. I had felt somehow that I had to go there, and that something was waiting for me there. I had already heard of the lakes and woods in southern Argentina, in the province of *Río Negro,* and the very special energy that surrounded this place.

When my friend Marian knew that I was planning a trip to the south, she referred me to this friend of hers, who ran a hotel with her family in San Carlos de Bariloche, near a lake called *Nahuel Huapi.* In March 2009, I made my first visit to Bariloche, and met the hotel owner; I stayed at her hotel and we became good friends. The visit was brief, as I could only afford a few days off from my work, but the experience of entering the woods and feeling the power of the mountains in the south was magical. There was an eerie, otherworldly feel about the place, and I felt the presence of the local elementals while I was there. Aqualead fit in perfectly in this scenery, considering the strong connection the local people had to the *Duendes*, a Spanish term referring to *Gnomes*. Figurines of Gnomes and Fairies were seen everywhere in artisan souvenir shops and craft stores in the small town.

My next trip away from Buenos Aires was to Bariloche a second time, in October 2009. This time I stayed longer, and I had more time to spend with my friend at the hotel. During my travels to Bariloche, I also met Patricio, who was a student and friend of Andrés. He later became the first Aqualead Master in Bariloche, and one of the directors of the Aqualead Society in Argentina. Other directors include Claudio in Buenos Aires and Liliana in Rosario, Santa Fé, as well as numerous regional representatives of the Aqualead Society. It seems that the energy expanded through travelling and reaching out to more remote and isolated areas.

While I was living in Buenos Aires, I had started taking Kung Fu classes, in order to learn something new and learn how to direct my energy in a new and challenging way. One of my classmates at the school where I trained was originally from the province of Córdoba, and told me about a friend he knew who ran a spiritual retreat in the mountains near Capilla del Monte. I had told him about my energy work and Aqualead; he became interested and eventually told his friends about it. It was around June of 2009, when I received an email from the owner of *Refugio Paso a Luz* in Capilla del Monte, inviting me to teach Aqualead to a group of people at their centre. She said in the message that there were a group of about 20 people who were interested. My first reaction to this unexpected invitation was that of fear and intimidation. I had never gone to Córdoba before, and I did not know these people at all. Also, I had never taught such a large group of people in my life. After some reflection, and a fair amount of hesitation, I responded to her and said I was open to the idea.

It was finally established, after a few months of emailing back and forth, that I would travel to Capilla del Monte in November 2009 to teach Aqualead. Due to the large group of students, I asked a friend of mine and Aqualead Master if she would come along for this trip, and help out with the classes; she accepted. We started out from the Retiro bus terminal, and travelled to the mountainous countryside of Córdoba, in November. Once at the bus station at Capilla del Monte, we waited for some time, and soon the owner's husband came to pick us up and drive us to their spiritual refuge, near *Ongamira.* This area, which is on *cerro Pajarillo*, is not far from the famed *cerro Uritorco*, where there have been many UFO sightings and reported close contacts with extraterrestrials. Many visitors came to this area in order to meditate, practise energy work and simply camp near this area, filled with this mystical energy.

We arrived at the spiritual centre, and were greeted by many people sitting in the house, on their small farm property in the mountains. Soon, the first Aqualead class was taught outside, near a stream cascading through some rocks. The students gathered and sat on rocks and logs, around me near the edge of the water, pens and notepads in hand. The outdoors was peaceful and fully reflected the spirit of Aqualead, while connecting to nature. They were a group of about 18 people, and many of them were family members of the owners who came from Rosario, Santa Fé. Thanks to my previous experiences teaching other healing modalities, I found my first two years of adaptation in Buenos Aires crucial, and I quickly realized that I was being prepared, in order to be able to teach my classes entirely in Spanish. Without this new language skill, teaching in these remote areas where no English was spoken would have been impossible. After I gave the initial lecture about Aqualead and taught the symbols, which everyone had on the handouts provided for them, I divided the group in half, and I gave attunements to one half of the group, while my friend gave attunements to the other half of the group. Everything worked out beautifully and the class atmosphere was suited for all ages. Soon, the entire class practised Aqualead on themselves and on one another, and we all sent energy at a distance. The change in energy in the entire place was obvious. It was a huge opportunity for me to be able to work with such amazing and trusting people, considering they had never met me before, and I was a foreigner in their country. Everything worked out of faith and trust, and working from this angle, nothing ever went wrong.

The next day, we continued with the Aqualead level II class. People were introduced to the symbols and, after the attunement, we were all sending distant healing, from the centre of Argentina. At the end of the class, I asked the group how they felt about doing the Aqualead Master level the next day, since my friend and I had to go back to Buenos Aires the next day in the afternoon. I explained to them that this was a lot of energy and information, on such a short basis. However, there was a feeling of urgency regarding learning this energy. There were recurring issues concerning droughts and forest fires in the area while we were there. After asking them who wanted to do the Master class, everyone in the group raised their hand; so I prepared the class for the next day. The rest of the day was spent either hiking in the mountains for some, or resting near the small cascading river while sitting in the sun, like I did. This area had a fascinating, otherworldly energy, as their small farm property sat in the middle of arid mountains. The walls of their house were adorned with surreal paintings of space ships, ascended masters and beams of light descending from the sky. An extension added to their house had glass bottles embedded within the cement walls, allowing daylight to come through. Crystals were embedded in the cement floor. The eerie atmosphere in this place made one want to sit down, and meditate on the spot.

The following morning was the Aqualead Master class, to a group of now 17 people. The group was again divided in two, and I attuned half of the class, while my helper attuned the other half of the group. The energy filled the room as the attunements were given. It was an amazing experience to be initiating so many Aqualead Masters all at once. It was even more rewarding interacting with a group of people that was so open to the rest of the universe. Aqualead was truly ready to spread outward. The students in the class then paired up and they practised Aqualead attunements. It seems as though they all had done it before. By the time we had all left, there now were Aqualead Masters in Córdoba province, and in Rosario, Santa Fé. These first Masters we initiated during those three days would begin many lineages of Aqualead, spreading throughout the provinces of Argentina.

My next significant travel in Argentina took place in January 2010, when I travelled to *Puerto Iguazu*, in the province of Misiones. I went there on vacation from work, and felt the need to go there and connect with the waters of the impressive Iguazu Falls, in the northern part of the country. I arrived alone by bus to the town of Puerto Iguazu, and walked a short distance to a hotel, where I felt drawn into entering. The owner was friendly, talkative and quickly set up a room for me. I did not yet realize my luck, as this was tourist high season (January is summertime in Argentina), and hotel rooms were typically impossible to find. What was more amazing is that at the hotel where I stayed, I befriended a couple from Mexico, who were staying there with their children. After a brief chat, I mentioned Aqualead and they became right away interested in learning it. This is how, during the brief time I stayed there, I ended up teaching all three levels of Aqualead to both of them. They became the first Aqualead Masters originally from Mexico.

I visited Iguazu National Park, and walked among the falls. I sent much Aqualead energy to those waters, and connecting to the power of the water there was a memorable experience. It was interesting to connect with the roaring white water, and watch these gigantic pillars of water crashing down, only a few feet away from me. I could also feel the hidden presence of elemental beings nearby, which guarded this powerful place. These falls are shared between the border of Argentina and Brazil; the Paraguayan border is also nearby. Later that year I made a last visit to Canada from Buenos Aires in December 2010, and I slowly began moving some of my belongings back home.

After my definitive return back to Canada in June 2011, the energy had me travelling abroad again. In September 2012, I travelled to Reykjavik, Iceland, to teach Aqualead through my friend whom I had met in Buenos Aires, while I was living there. I then participated in a holistic fair in Mosfellsbaer, near Reykjavik, on my first visit. It seemed the energy wanted to expand itself in different places; on my second trip to Iceland, I was able to visit the island far more extensively thanks to my friends, from the south to the westfjords. I later travelled to New Jersey, United States, in October 2012, to share Aqualead with groups of new friends and students, after connecting with a friend and Reiki Master who resides there.

CHAPTER III:

HEALING AND MANIFESTATION

i. More information comes through

The Aqualead Program started out with only four symbols and a limited amount of information. I always thought that the modality would remain the same. However, this proved to be wrong. As of May 2009, the program expanded and more information was added, which is something I did not expect. My channelling work continued and advanced furthermore, to a higher level. I was at work again on the evening of May 14th, when I received the nudge to draw more symbols. I was not sure if these symbols were to be used for the Aqualead system; regardless, I simply followed the energy's lead. Over a span of a few days, I drew a series of five additional symbols, each with a name. Almost simultaneously, I received far more detailed information about all the new and existing symbols of Aqualead. The new symbols channelled were not related to water, however greatly expanded the range of healing energy work that a practitioner and Master could perform. These symbols were sent to me by my masters; however, I did not feel any angel present this time. The first of these new symbols I channelled constituted for me another turning point in my life; this symbol, which I will call the *transformation symbol*, seemed to me by far the most powerful of all the symbols in the Aqualead system. This symbol was so strong that my first thought was to integrate this symbol at the Master level.

Later, however, my guides instructed me to incorporate it at the second practitioner level, so more people could learn and use it. This transformation symbol proved to be, in my opinion, the most important and influential symbol in Aqualead.

Other symbols were also added to the levels, which meant a student had more than one symbol to work with, at each level. This brought on a huge shift in the practice, learning and teaching of Aqualead. Practitioners could expand their range of healing in other ways than just focusing on water. It felt to me as though we had just received an upgrade. Soon after studying and incorporating these symbols in the Aqualead Program, I contacted all the Masters and practitioners and briefed them. Fortunately, there was no need for any further attunements. All existing practitioners and Masters were already attuned to the frequency of these symbols; it was only a matter of transmitting the information. Back then, it was easy to trace back all the people who had Aqualead. I always maintained a record of all my classes and students, along with dates. There were relatively few of them at the time. It was good timing also, because this shift occurred before my first visit to Capilla del Monte.

Around this time, I had moved from the apartment in the barrio of Almagro, to my very own apartment in the cosmopolitan neighbourhood of *Belgrano*, on Cabildo Street. This move occurred roughly a month before all this new information arrived, which meant for me much more freedom in my range of action with Aqualead. I was now living alone in my tiny bachelor apartment, and was able to have visitors in my own space, which I could not do before. This meant I had my own classroom, and was able to teach Aqualead students in my home. My small flat then became an Aqualead school. I do remember actually channelling the transformation symbol in my apartment late in the evening, after coming home from work; I had already scribbled the information and the name of the symbol on some paper, while sitting at work.

With the use of these new symbols, the range of personal and environmental healing was enhanced, and now enabled us to work on different aspects of healing the Earth. Some of these new aspects of the energy introduced were the areas of agriculture and plant growth, the transformation and dispelling of negative energies and animal awareness and communication, as well as alternative forms of energy implemented on the Master level. We now had a total of nine symbols. The new presence of the transformation symbol had an intense effect and seemed to have the ability to release and expose any kind of negative situation or energy, and release it out into the open. The symbol seemed to bring order out of the chaos. This new tool seemed perfectly adapted and needed for our world, so saturated with lower energies and violence. What was also perfect about this significant new symbol was that its healing range was not specifically limited to healing water and nature. It could be applied to human society or to institutions, such as governments, companies or schools. They could also be used on ideas or ideologies, such as racism, or any kind of negative situation or form of injustice, which did not necessarily have a natural origin. With the arrival of this new transformation symbol, I felt that the healing with Aqualead had been taken one step further; and it seemed to me that we were all up to the challenge. Aqualead was definitely carrying us to the next step, and to the next level of dimension.

Soon after, I met with my friend Marian, and she had expressed a desire for us Aqualead Masters to gather at her house and spend a day to practise and incorporate the energy of each one of the nine symbols. I felt that was an excellent idea. One day, a group of eight of us gathered at her house, and we went through each one of the symbols, and at each symbol we would focus on the elements that were attributed to each symbol. It appeared as though we were conducting an arts and crafts workshop. However, this allowed the energy of Aqualead to express its creativity and colours to us. We put music, essential oils, incense, crystals, flowers and other of the elements attributed that could be added to each symbol. This was a worthwhile process, and I thank Marian for having had such a great idea. It helped us feel the energy of each one of these symbols, and ground them into us, in our Aqualead practice. This is how Aqualead was meant to grow and expand. The process was enlightening and enriching for all of us at the personal and creative level. At this point, with the amount of information and knowledge that we had received, I thought this completed the modality. However, there was still more knowledge coming.

A holistic fair was later held at Marian's place, where different people could bring their works and share with the rest of the community. The fair included crafts, crystals, massage therapists and vegetarian food. I showed Aqualead at this expo and the success was great; this was Aqualead's first public appearance. I also taught the first level of Aqualead to a group of students, during the event. It created more connections, and some people I met at this event later became Aqualead Masters. One of these new Masters created more connections with other new students; this is how I eventually met friends Claudio, Roberto and many others who showed up in my tiny apartment to learn Aqualead. Claudio later became a prominent and influential figure in Aqualead, as the director of the Aqualead Society in Buenos Aires, and greatly assisted me in producing official Aqualead manuals in Spanish while I was there.

ii. The return of the Unicorns

I never thought I would ever have a connection with Unicorns. However, Aqualead proved otherwise. In December 2009, another wave of symbols came to me. I channelled six additional symbols, which were to be called the *Unicorn symbols*. I had no idea what to do with these, and I imagined these symbols were to be kept to myself. According to my guides, these symbols healed mainly at the human, emotional level. They were to be introduced to the Aqualead Masters only, as an extension to their range of healing in a session. Only Masters could learn these symbols, and they were already attuned to them through one of the Master symbols. They simply needed to be introduced to them, and know their uses. Even though I was newly acquainted with elemental beings, Unicorns were beings that were fairly unknown to me. It was the actual channelling process that introduced me to them, and to their apparent past history on Earth.

I discovered through these energies that not only do Unicorns truly exist but also that they are living beings. Only, like other elementals, they live in the same time frame as us, however, they belong to a much higher dimension than our own. There is no obvious evidence of the previous existence of Unicorns on Earth, but I was always fascinated by the numerous images of Unicorns either seen on French medieval tapestries, medieval art or appearing in European and British heraldry and coat of arms. There somehow seemed to be some awareness or knowledge of them during that period; were artists back then inspired by an unseen source? If Unicorns really did exist in this world at some point, have they become extinct? And if so, what happened to them? I found it peculiar and interesting that I would be sent these new symbols, corresponding to the healing vibration of these elevated beings, already known to this world since long ago.

And here I was, being told by my masters that even though these magical beings are still considered legend in our world, they too had healing abilities we could harness. These symbols were rays of this vibration of Light, and by working with these symbols, we were tapping directly into this highly pure, innocent and sensitive vibration of the Unicorns. Regardless of whether one believes in the existence and presence of Unicorns, I do know that these symbols worked; and one who had the ability to use them could deal with a wide range of emotions, such as anger, guilt, shame, grief and fear. And I do recall channelling one of the symbols that evening, which just so happened to look like a Unicorn, and feeling a sudden surge of emotion, which felt like anger and frustration, as I was frantically trying to make out what this symbol was meant to be like. It felt as though the Unicorn wanted to jump out of the paper at me, which in fact it did.

What was remarkable with the Unicorn symbols is that they were specifically addressed to deal with human issues. It seemed the environmental healing was already dealt with in Aqualead. These symbols were excellent to use in a wide range of emotional issues, such as depression, stress and different kinds of emotional trauma. One symbol proved to be excellent for dealing with sexual abuse, both for the victim and the perpetrator. Another one of the Unicorn symbols was ideal for resolving conflicts, helping manage anger, frustration and rage. Another symbol had the ability to deal with genetic problems and issues transmitted through parental genes. It was interesting to see what these symbols could do, and how they functioned and healed. We were all intrigued and amazed at how effective this intense emotional healing worked, through working with the Unicorn symbols.

As with the added symbols, these too were introduced and offered to the Masters. Not all Aqualead Masters have learned the Unicorn symbols; learning and using them is purely optional. However, they enhance the range of the healing performed on a person, and the person receiving the healing greatly benefited as a result. The implementation of the six Unicorn symbols did not imply adding a new level to the Aqualead Program. Aqualead still remained with the same three levels, but the Unicorn symbols were considered an addition for the Masters who were interested in acquiring the symbols and applying them in their practice.

iii. Working with the Elves

Ever since my first encounter with them during my second visit to Canada, I always felt the elementals' presence with me, everywhere I went. I always felt accompanied and well protected at all times. This connection with them enabled me to relate more to them on a personal level, with respect to their way of life and their closeness to nature. These elementals were wise, forgiving and generally compassionate towards the human race; and my close contact with them enabled me to appreciate those characteristics. They too were familiar with healing nature and animals, as well as clearing negative energy and holding the space. These beings struck me as being natural healers and manifestors; their high vibration of energy enabled them to work with the elements and bring in new situations that seemed unthinkable. They appeared to be masters of abundance and reminded me of the generosity of the universe itself. The Elves reminded me of grass effortlessly growing from the ground or the sun shining endlessly, regardless of the number of beings benefiting from its rays. I felt very little concern for sustenance or prosperity in their presence. And up until this day, I remain with this peaceful and secure feeling, knowing that the universe always provides. This is only one of the valuable lessons the Elves have taught me over a period of time. I am not sure if Aqualead energy has attracted them, or if perhaps their presence increased the effect of the energy. I am also uncertain whether they were related to those same beings from which the energy was sent to me. However, they clearly seemed to me as having a strong purifying effect on their surroundings and on others, which is what Aqualead also does. There is a close similarity between the two energies.

As with supporting and protecting nature, Aqualead also offered a higher energy vibration that appealed to the elementals and their environment. Fairies became more clearly visible by those who had Aqualead, and it seems that the energy, especially at the second level, attracted them towards the sender. The number of Fairy sightings among my students dramatically increased with the use and practise of Aqualead. Some of my friends, who are sensitive healers and Aqualead Masters, could perceive the presence of the elemental beings in my apartment or around me as we worked with the energy.

The Elves' increased presence in our world sends us a powerful message about the importance of connecting with the Earth and the necessity to live our lives more in harmony and with respect towards the planet. This notion also applies to all animals, both domestic and wild. Another important message from these wise beings is the importance of acknowledging, respecting and honouring trees, like they do.

iv. The river within

Over time, I felt guided by the energy to incorporate and reinforce meditation in the practice of Aqualead. I felt meditating would help practitioners and Masters deepen their practice of Aqualead, at each one of the levels. Another thing which was later reinforced, thanks to my Elven friends, was the emphasis on the connection with the presence and the energy of trees. Spending time in nature in the presence of these tall majestic beings was very helpful in the practice of Aqualead, and served as a reminder of the reason why Aqualead was here. Meditation is a basic skill in many spiritual practices, such as yoga. It is universal and allows the practitioner to clear their energy and their mind, which creates a favourable energy space in which the energy work is better conducted. Meditation improves one's skills as a healer and enables one to sharpen their minds, and circulate their energy in order for it to balance itself through the body. I found that implementing meditation in the Aqualead Program was most helpful and useful for all practitioners and Masters.

I also discovered through the energy, and through its very high frequency, the importance of remaining grounded while working with Aqualead. This was most crucial to practise at the Master level, where the four symbols are very strong and are more related to manifesting and giving attunements. I almost always emphasize this point in class to my students; especially before they begin practising. I always turned the focus of the healing session on the ankles and feet, where the actual grounding occurs.

This was most important so practitioners remained grounded and connected to the present moment, while doing this very high energy work. Students are always grounded at the end of the Aqualead attunement in the class, for this reason.

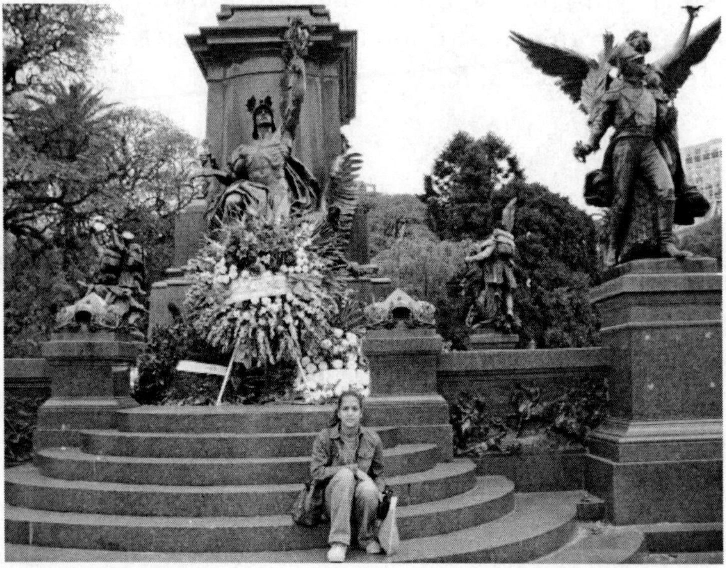

1. Just arrived in Buenos Aires, in September 2006; I was still new to the capital city, and adapting to my surroundings.

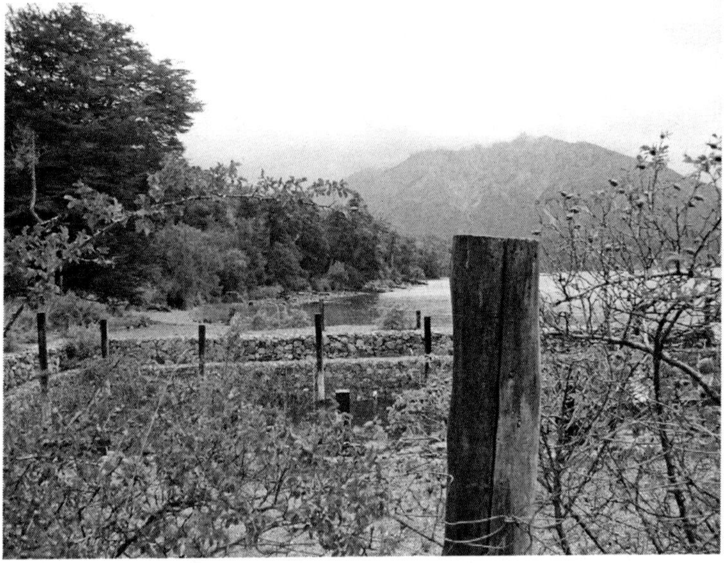

2. Visit to Bariloche, in the Argentine province of Rio Negro, in March 2009. Bariloche became a permanent home for Aqualead.

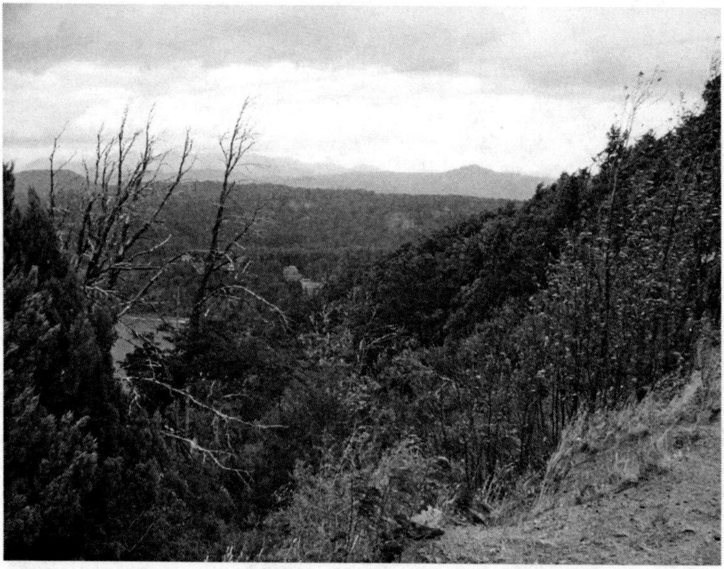

3. *Parque Nacional Llao Llao*, near Bariloche, Argentina.

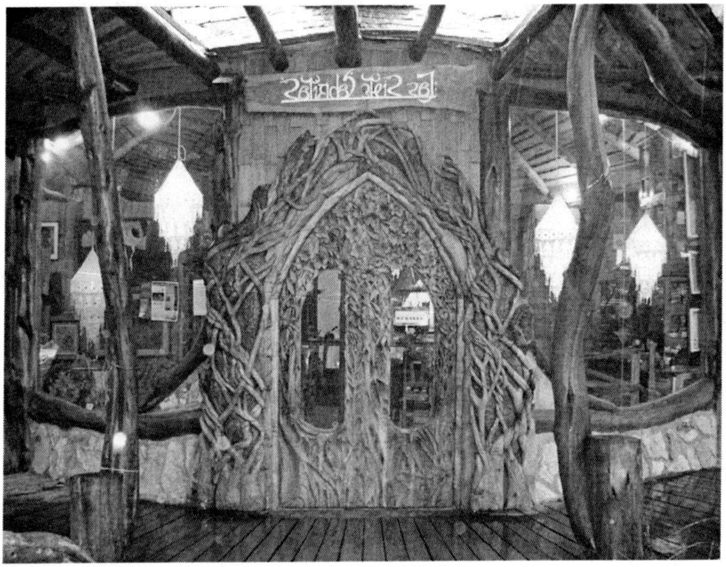

4. An *Elvish door* on a shop in *Colonia Suiza*, near Bariloche, in southern Argentina.

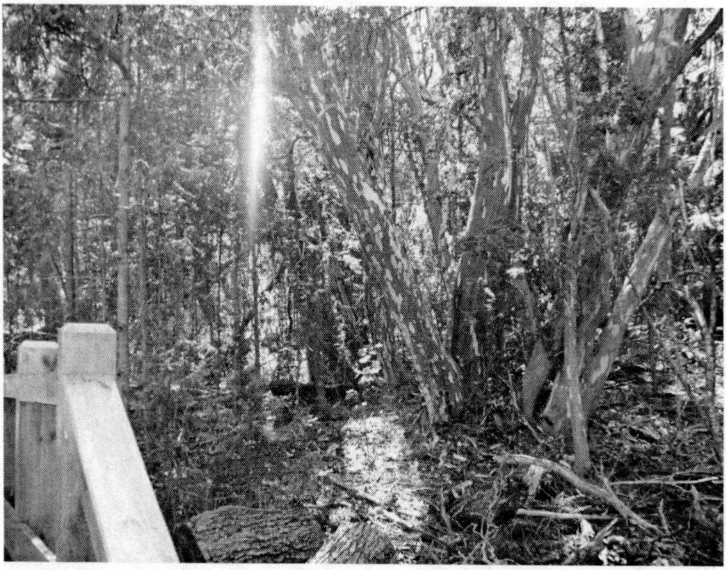

5. *Bosque Arrayanes*, on *Lago Nahuel Huapi.* These trees have a unique appearance, and many *globes of light* appeared in photos I took in these woods.

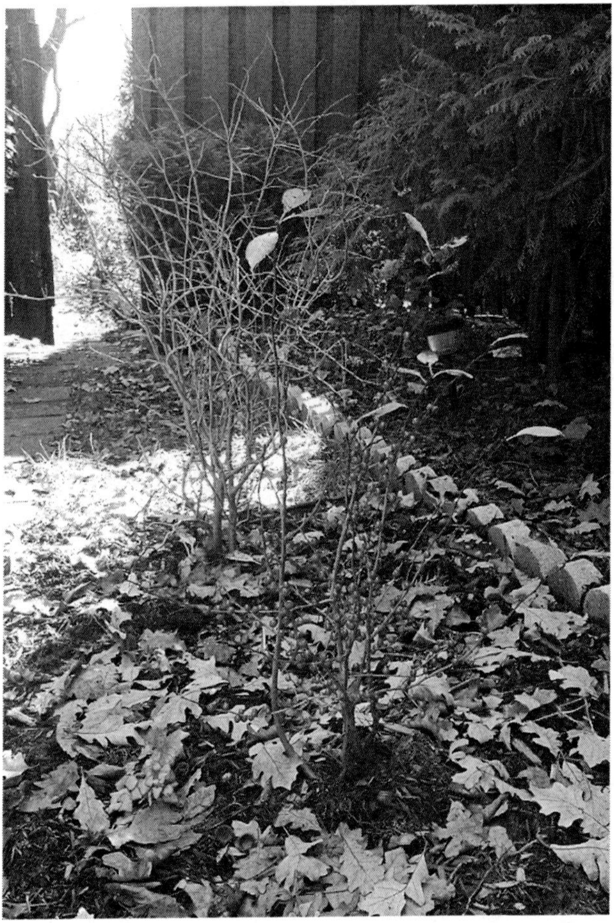

6. Aqualead has a noticeable effect here in Canada, in every living being.

PART II

PRACTISING AND TEACHING AQUALEAD

CHAPTER IV:

THE EARTH AND THE UNIVERSE

i. From one ocean to the next

The practice of Aqualead is in essence just as important as teaching it, if not more. Aqualead is an energy that has its own will; it carries its intention to heal and cleanse water and the entire planet. However, in order to get here, or to be applied to something, it must be directed and channelled through the hands of a healer. The more Aqualead is practised and sent remotely at a distance, the more Aqualead energy is present in this world. Once funnelled into this dimension, the energy remains here and begins to do its work. This would explain why it felt so urgent at the very beginning to start teaching Aqualead to willing students, and enable them to teach it so early. The energy simply wanted to get out there, and begin clearing the contamination in many different places. We needed to start initiating this process as soon as possible. Being unique in its own right, I understood from this energy that it has also served me as a guide and a teacher. I therefore had to listen to it, and follow its cue. This is the reason why it seemed inevitable for me to let this energy go outward, in order for it to do its work. The energy travelled not only through me but also through other practitioners, Masters, and their students. Through some of my students, other new practitioners and Masters appeared as the modality spread; very soon there were more of us practising Aqualead.

We realized we could send Aqualead to everything and anything, whether it was to a forest fire, the poaching of endangered animals or a domestic dispute. The range of Aqualead practice broadened: some practitioners and students of Aqualead began incorporating Aqualead in their own energy healing work, by combining it with other healing/holistic methods such as Reiki, massage, reflexology, aromatherapy and yoga. Some Aqualead Masters began applying Aqualead on cancer patients, or to those having other severe chronic illnesses. Some people have asked me if it was possible to treat patients suffering from other such illnesses with Aqualead, and I have said to them: *"Yes, of course. Try it."* An important aspect of Aqualead energy is that its purpose is only to heal and create changes in order to produce a positive healing effect. It cannot be used with negative intent and this energy, as strong as it may be, cannot cause harm or aggravate the illness of a person. What it may do, however, is produce strong releasing symptoms, as the body begins to release energies and toxins; this discomfort is temporary, despite being unpleasant, and a greater feeling of well-being follows after the cleansing is complete.

The energy has proven to be versatile and applicable to all aspects of human life. Aqualead has also been practised in pregnancy, childbirth and to patients recovering from surgery, with some positive outcomes. This of course *does not guarantee* that Aqualead will completely cure any of these illnesses; however, there is a possibility and hope that somehow it can bring some positive changes, and provide these patients with some relief and support. Aqualead opens a new range of possibilities in energy work, due to the fact that it heals and changes the water in every cell of a person's body. Water constitutes over 70% of a person's body mass; once exposed to the energy, it can therefore release a considerable amount of toxins from the body. The more we have practised Aqualead, the more we have learned and acquired new insights into its practice and the support it has provided to others, not only at the physical level but also at the emotional and mental levels. Discovering the practice of Aqualead on a multitude of issues and situations was an adventure in healing in itself, however, not in a reckless kind of way, but rather as being guided onto a new and challenging journey. This energy is indeed a teacher to those who are open to receiving its wisdom.

The energy of Aqualead is still new, and its high vibration has been known to create a certain shock with its surroundings. This reaction is normal until the local environment adjusts to the higher vibration. This entails the release of old or lower energies. This is generally how the healing process will occur. This healing crisis may not only occur in the human body; this can also occur in situations where a formidable amount of energy is released, seemingly aggravating the situation. I have warned my students before about this process, especially when teaching the transformation symbol. When it is used, the situation will release its unbalance or negativity, exposing it to be seen in full view. This release will often bring on a crisis, and through this crisis, a higher level of order can be established. This is the reason why Aqualead may initially seem to intensify an already existing situation of crisis. However, this aggravation is temporary, as there were probably underlying hidden issues, such as lower energies or other factors that needed to be exposed to the light beforehand.

Due to the fact that Aqualead is a subtle healing energy, as opposed to the more common energies the world already knows, such as electricity or solar power, it makes it awkward to prove scientifically that this energy works and is useful in modern society. Subtle energies are like colours: they are not visible on their own until they are applied to a physical object. Only then, the colour becomes visible as *red* or *blue*. Hence, it would be difficult to measure the effectiveness of Aqualead by itself in scientific research, or on any particular physical instrument. Up until now, no tests have been performed on water, before and after being treated with Aqualead. If someone is willing to perform this experiment, I would be more than eager to see the results, if any. But on my part, I will not take any initiative towards that direction, because I find this irrelevant and unnecessary for me to know that Aqualead does have an effect. And analyzing water samples would not, in my mind, further validate or measure the success of Aqualead's healing work.

This is an energy I have learned to trust, from its beginning. And when I look back at the entire channelling process and how my friends and colleagues so eagerly became involved, I am not concerned about the need to back Aqualead energy's validity with scientific research or special instruments. Those who have shown an interest in learning Aqualead were truly ready and prepared to do so. Sceptics, who may be uncomfortable with the idea behind this new energy, have simply refrained from coming forward. To me, it is a matter of *being ready* to embark on this new journey, and also a question of personal timing. I do believe there is a time for everything in a person's life, and in order to begin learning Aqualead, the timing for that person must be right. It is all related to being receptive to the universe and following the signs, as well as the guidance which is sent to us.

Aqualead is here to teach us many things: to review and question everything we have learned in the past, about our ways of life, our consumption habits, the way we treat one another within the human race, and especially other species. This is how, at times, I feel that Aqualead is not just a new healing tool but also a new way of thinking about ourselves, almost as a movement of change. It seems, from the use and practice of this energy, that a new philosophy and lifestyle are emanating, having close similarities with aboriginal ways of life and even at times, some elements of *shamanism.* Perhaps through the use of Aqualead, something old will re-emerge from the past that we all believed to be extinct. I see Aqualead as a new way for us to redefine ourselves. This energy is holding up the mirror in front of us and this world, not only to show us our flaws but also to indicate where the change and the focus of the healing needs to take place.

All the issues around the world we are currently facing, such as violence, corruption, sexual abuse, pollution, deforestation and animal cruelty, are becoming more visible, obvious and therefore more disturbing. I have noticed this with people around me practising Aqualead or becoming Aqualead Masters, how at the personal level in their life some major changes have occurred. Some Masters underwent a deep personal transformation, other have encountered changes in their relationships, such as a separation; other people have moved or relocated, while others experienced a major change in their habits and lifestyle, in a positive way. Many experienced a series of healing symptoms, as the energy seemed to purge something inside them outwards; however, after the crisis they became healthier and stronger than ever.

The practice of Aqualead is mainly hands-on healing. However, one does not always need the contact of hands in order to send the energy. Energy always follows intention. Aqualead is usually practised by placing the hands directly over certain energy centres in the human body (called *chakras*). Not all chakras are treated in Aqualead, and I discovered there is a reason for this. For instance, we skip the crown chakra because through the sixth chakra, called the *Third Eye*, the energy enters and does all the work in the upper area of the body and the brain. The Third Eye is connected to the pineal gland, which is a very important organ related to meditation, spirituality and consciousness. It is at this level Aqualead wants to focus the work in a person at the level of awareness and consciousness. The third eye is also related to clairvoyance, and the ability to see what the physical eyes cannot perceive. It is related to seeing the truth behind dissimulation, and dissipating illusions. It is interesting to see that through working at such a high level of energy in a person, the energy will heal them by increasing insight and help the person discern the reality behind the issues they are confronted with.

This is another important aspect of healing, which is not only relieving the symptoms of the illness and changing the issue for a more positive outcome but also for the person to understand the *reason why* that issue is there. Every illness or problem in one's life carries a message and provides clues to a person as to what direction one needs to take in life. This also applies to relationships with others. Healing an issue often means understanding the underlying message behind it, and then integrating these lessons into one's own consciousness. Then, the person is released from this pattern and is able to move forward, as the blockage has been removed. The consciousness surrounding the issue is just as important as the healing session performed or sent remotely at a distance. Much of the healing work done with Aqualead revolves around this aspect. When we are able to understand *why* these diseases occur and their reasons for being there in the first place, it opens a new healing space from which we can cooperate, and prevent this disease from reoccurring.

ii. Crossing dimensions

Aqualead is a healing energy of a higher dimension than this one; I consider it an energy of the *fifth dimension.* Not only is it felt intuitively, it can also be felt physically as it is practised, and through the types of changes it brings. It is noticed in its strength and character. It is a lively energy that simply feels like nothing else in this world, which brings more healing possibilities and manifestation. The different spiritual dimensions expand as follows: the *third dimension* is a denser level of consciousness. It is focused on the physical and material states of being; it is also a space that creates a static duality between the concepts of *good* and *evil.* In the *fourth dimension*, we begin to see these two polarities clashing, as we strive towards a higher level of Light. This level sees a shift and a greater ability to transcend these lower, darker energies. At the *fifth dimension,* we reach a higher level of Light forms and stellar beings. We enter a more *cosmic* level: there is no more fear, only oneness. This is the level where we encounter greater Light, love and the absence of physical suffering.

The fact that Aqualead feels stronger has been unanimously observed among those who practise it and can compare it with other healing energies. It seems that this energy is here to precipitate deep changes; however, this change is necessary at the planetary level, meaning our relationship with the Earth, and forces us to question how we treat it. And it seems that we are achieving this with a new energy that is from beyond, and was clearly sent to us by an outside intelligence. I also know that Aqualead is here to spark evolution on this planet, and among ourselves. This evolution of the human race will be impossible unless we change our relationship with the Earth and animals. This crossing and shifting of dimensions occurs in the progression of the Aqualead Program, after the second level of Aqualead is completed. The fifth dimension is recognizable by the apparition of energy portals; these are doorways which serve as passages and allow the safe encounter with higher energies.

The fifth dimension works at this level: we begin thinking beyond the scope of ourselves and our own personal interests. We are now asking ourselves: *what can help us evolve as a species? What hinders or blocks our evolution? What needs to change from within us?* Aqualead takes us to that level, due to its nature. We also begin thinking further: *Are all species on Earth coexisting in a peaceful, balanced state? If not, why?* What is also particular about Aqualead is that the healing is not only centred on human beings. Aqualead addresses itself equally to trees, plant life and to all animal species, not only to household pets. No one is forgotten or left behind, even if breaking this barrier involves exposing painful truths. This is the path Aqualead is asking us to take; it is a difficult challenge, asking us to let go of our daily commodities and forcing us to question our habits. This is a difficult task to undertake at the personal level, yet we need this personal confrontation in order to see what is limiting us. Aqualead is telling us to begin pondering ourselves as a human race, and ask ourselves if our society and way of life are not creating victims. This is what Aqualead wants to expose and heal, therefore, pushing forward the limits of our awareness, and of our *comfort zone*. And this energy seems to want to perform this type of transition quickly, without delay; it seems the energy is pushing us and preparing us for a radical change.

After a few years now working with Aqualead and teaching it, I have developed a deep respect for it and I am always ever so grateful for this gift in the world and in my life. However, the energy is revealing that there is still much work to be done. The very idea of stopping human damage on the Earth, and eventually reversing its effect seems like a daunting and far-fetched undertaking. But, I believe this is what Aqualead is here to help us achieve. The message I have received from the unexpected arrival of this new form of healing is that *everything and anything is possible*. However, it will take time. I have noticed that energy healing work is often done gradually; most of the time there are no instant overnight results. The effect of the healing and subsequent releasing is the equivalent of peeling an onion: there is an element of timing involved, and it may become an exercise in patience. The actual healing, or *cure*, may be achieved only in a matter of years. Assisting the planet in its transformation may very well take centuries: this would be done in conjunction with helping balance the elements of nature, and reconciling the immense conflict created between human societies and nature. Of course, the planet does not have centuries to wait in this state; and with these alarming issues caused by human activity and wars, there is a greater need for urgent action, and more people practising and teaching Aqualead.

Now we are contemplating a new path, a very challenging one, for the growing Aqualead communities worldwide, working with the new energy. We now have a new way of breaking down old and obsolete structures and, through the chaos, establishing a new higher order. This rapid shifting of dimensions is allowing us to achieve just that. Such a shift will also help confront and break through the human ego and selfishness, so we can see the true path that lies before us without becoming biased by self-interest. This way, it is my hope that in the future we will reach a higher level of peace, justice and love, as well as a genuine harmony with the Earth and nature.

iii. The Aqualead students

Without Aqualead students, there would be neither Aqualead practitioners nor any eventual Masters at all. I feel that of all the energy work I have done, nothing brings me more satisfaction than teaching the very first level, and transporting a new person through the threshold of Aqualead and the world of energy healing. The people coming to me to learn Aqualead could be anyone, coming from any type of background. Aqualead is available for everyone, coming from any walk of life; there are no prerequisites for learning the first level of Aqualead. Being free of charge, students do not need to be wealthy, or from a higher social class in order to access its benefits. All and everyone are welcome. I have taught highly trained and experienced healers; I have also taught complete beginners without any previous experience in energy healing work. And quite frankly, I have seen spectacular results in both types of students. What I have noticed in teaching this modality is the high number of students who promptly continued to the next level, reaching the Master level fairly fast. There seemed to never be any apprehension or hesitation in the newcomers I have taught. People seem to instinctively know that this energy healing is important, not to say urgent for some.

Working with students has always been a magical experience for me. I also found that Aqualead classes became a very bonding experience for all those who were present. People tended to join together, and maintain friendships after the class. Communities quickly formed either physically, or through groups in social media on the Internet. Many of the friends I have made in Argentina, and other parts of the world, were brought on by this energy and the work done with students in the class. There always seemed to be an atmosphere of trust and oneness with Aqualead. Perhaps the energy attracts people who are open to new things and are not afraid of change. It could be due to the fact that many people worldwide, not only healers, share a growing concern for the fate and future of this planet and animal welfare. In some of my Aqualead classes, these issues generated discussion among the students in the groups. What was surprising to me was how easily the topic of elemental beings came into the conversation. It seems that Aqualead serves as a reminder to people of a part of them they thought was forgotten or lost. Also, the Aqualead classes provided a safe space for student to share their experiences and beliefs in the elemental world, without the fear or embarrassment of being ridiculed.

iv. Sending energy worldwide

We have also arranged group healings, whether in person or remotely at a distance; we have sent energy all in unison, either to the oceans, the Amazon rainforest or a nearby river. As the new Aqualead symbols appeared, I extended the group healings into healing projects with Aqualead healing, such as *Aqualead for the Amazon*, and *Aqualead for Africa.* The project *Aqualead for the Amazon* focused on dealing with deforestation issues, endangered animals species and supporting aboriginal rights. Also, a huge amount of Aqualead healing was sent at a distance to the African continent, where I turned my focus towards human rights and the protection of women and children. We have also sent Aqualead energy to the oceans in the midst of oil spills, whale and dolphin hunting, corrupt governments and political upset. Some of us, including myself, have sent Aqualead energy to the entire world, or to the Earth on a mass global scale. The possibilities are endless. Often, the energy will direct the healer where it needs to be sent, and the healers will feel intuitively guided to perform healing or send distant healing to a particular issue. Since the purpose of this energy is to balance nature and also the life it supports, the energy seemed very drawn towards animal species and ecosystems, and has greatly focused its healing work there. Hopefully the notion of *peace on Earth* will be understood in a new light, and will extend to all life forms on Earth, not only as an exclusive right reserved for the human race.

Aqualead reminds us that we are one, and made of the same thing. The majority of the healing work done with Aqualead is focused on this aspect, which works in conjunction with healing water. My hope is that Aqualead will help bridge this gap between human activity and nature, and help the human race transcend its barriers. As we continue healing ourselves and the Earth, we continue transforming the structures in human societies, and transmuting negative energies all over the world. It is my hope that there will be a new balance between all life, and a clear understanding and respect for other species that are currently being enslaved. By sending Aqualead to the Earth and all oceans, I wish the same freedom for all species, as well as for our own.

CHAPTER V

THE PATH OF THE AQUALEAD MASTER

i. Teacher vs. Master

An Aqualead Master is a person who has completed the third level of Aqualead; this entails two skills they now possess: that of using and practising the Master symbols, and also the ability to teach and give Aqualead attunements. I have noticed that the majority of the very first students that I've taught completed all three levels and reached the Master level promptly. And this rapid progression throughout the levels was not coerced by me in any way. The Aqualead Master level is a unique path; not only does it enhance a practitioner's skill range and offer the possibility to teach, it also provides a new challenge as a personal and spiritual path, and as an exercise in detachment. This level of Aqualead is focused on the theme of *manifestation.* In the two practitioner levels, we have focused our energy on healing the Earth and water, the environment, animal species and human issues. All the wide range of the healing work is performed at the first and second levels of Aqualead.

When the student ventures into the Master level, the energy work takes on a different feel. We begin stepping outside of the scope of healing, and entering a new level of challenge and personal growth. This level demonstrates how we are meant to surpass our obstacles and limitations, in a safe and practical way. Many Aqualead Masters, however, may opt not to practise Aqualead at all; others will practise and do some healing work, while others may decide to take on the path of teaching. When a Master student completes the third level, they are told that teaching is *optional* and is not an obligation. Teaching is not for everyone; and even though a person can make an excellent Aqualead Master as a healer or practise it at the personal and spiritual levels, that person may not be suited to teach. I have known great Aqualead Masters who have never taught a class in their life. One does not need to be a teacher or have any experience teaching in order to internalize and fully understand the information and resonate with the energy. Being a Master requires one to *master* their own self, and the knowledge they have acquired; this process often requires time.

The essence of being an Aqualead Master begins with one's inner self, and the energy one carries. It is also a matter of intention. This new path is one of self-knowledge and purification. One cannot take on the world and begin healing others unless they are healed themselves and have completed the process of reviewing their life and their own past. Everything needs to be re-examined, throughout all the relationships encountered, past personal experiences, family background and childhood. It is a process of introspection, and allows one to re-assess their reasons for wanting to complete the third level of Aqualead. Practitioners who have the second level of Aqualead are encouraged to do this. First, they should review and fully know the information taught in the Aqualead Program. They need to memorize the symbols; I believe that a Master of any discipline, regardless of what it is, should know the information and be readily able to use it, practise it, demonstrate it and eventually teach it. This is knowledge that becomes innate and automatic. This is what mastering a discipline entails: it requires time, study, practise and self-discipline. This is something that is fundamental. Aqualead is a skill on the practical level that is learned, acquired and practised. When one reaches the Master level of Aqualead, one must be made aware of the responsibility it involves; even more so if they desire to teach it to the general public. This is why a self-review is important, as well as reviewing one's intentions, which will transpire in a class from the beginning.

Aqualead Masters are given a position of authority to a certain degree, if they begin dealing with the public and representing the energy modality to others. If a Master begins using his or her title to impress, manipulate others or to serve their own personal interests, the quality of practice and teaching is greatly lost. For this reason the cooperation of all is necessary, in order to keep the intention of Aqualead Masters pure in their behaviour and teaching. Masters are serving the Light and the greater interests of the Earth. Being a Master of any practice or discipline means showing respect towards others and the modality, and ultimately towards the students.

This is the reason why I emphasize preparation before the completion of this level. It should be treated with respect and undertaken with great care and awareness. With this amount of energy in their hands, Aqualead Masters are given a very wide range of skills and are granted a fair amount of power. It should be used wisely, with an attitude of gratitude, love, service and dedication towards the Earth. This is a very meaningful step one chooses to undertake. This is also the reason why new Masters need to wait and take time to fully integrate the energy from the Master training, and become fully knowledgeable of the energy itself before beginning to teach it to others. Great care must be taken to maintain the accuracy of the program, and also of the attunement procedure; there should be no modifications in that respect. Aqualead is not only a status and a modality but also a way of life.

This, however, does not mean that the Aqualead Masters become perfect and enlightened beings right away. The mastery of any skill requires time and often a lifetime of practise. And in most cases, it is an opportunity to learn, grow and practise humility. However, teaching Aqualead does require acute knowledge of the modality and the understanding and respect for the Aqualead Program, in order to avoid any inconsistencies and discrepancies. Also, it is important for the public approaching a Master that this person be reliable in delivering the energy and the information accurately. Generally, many Aqualead practitioners become Masters; however, fewer of them may opt to teach it.

I have added here a series of questions an Aqualead practitioner at the second level should ask themselves before undertaking the third Master level course. I feel it may be helpful for some, in order to assess their knowledge, thoughts and intentions on their advancement in their Aqualead training.

Questionnaire for Aqualead level II practitioners wanting to undertake the Master level:

- Do I feel ready to take this course?
- Can I draw all the symbols correctly, as well as write their names?
- Have I memorized the symbols?
- Am I practising Aqualead enough, or sending distant healing on occasion?
- Do I fully understand Aqualead energy, its purpose and its nature?
- What are my intentions as an Aqualead Master? Do I want to teach?
- Have I waited at least four months after completing Aqualead level II?

ii. Slowing down

After Aqualead was first channelled, I understood from my masters that there had to be a minimum wait time of 24 hours between attunements. Despite this, it was clearly understood to me that before undertaking the Master level, students should wait a longer time period than that. This wait time was never clearly defined between the second level and the third, but after a rapid proliferation of the numbers of Aqualead Masters, I felt guided and compelled to implement a specific time limit, in order to reduce the exaggerated number of Aqualead Masters either being taught badly or teaching too quickly. At this point I have added a four-month wait period between the second and third levels of Aqualead, and this helped slow some people down. It seemed to have improved the quality of the teaching and the general focus on quality rather than just quantity. It is more rewarding to learn a modality slowly and take the time to absorb it, and take even more time before teaching it; the wait is more than likely worthwhile. This also implemented a sense of awareness and consciousness, which comes with the desire to undertake the Master level of such a modality. This was a part of the learning and development process that Aqualead has brought to all of us. The learning and growth continue onward.

Another element that struck me about the Master level is the greater amount of meditation it seemed to embrace. I found myself spending more time in meditation with these symbols, while the symbols of the two practitioner levels seemed more proactive and aimed towards tackling the outside world. I found that the Master level brought on a much deeper insight, not only in the healing work done but also in terms of detaching myself from others and becoming more withdrawn in reflection, almost in the form of a personal retreat. In the space of contemplation and observation I found myself in, I was then able to observe the world, human activity, plants and animals and understand things on a much deeper level. What the energy of the Aqualead Master symbols echoed to me was the preparation for the coming of a new world and a new Earth. This new society we would establish would be completely different from the one we live in now, which is currently destructive. I saw a world of peace, where trees were honoured and respected; animals were revered as wise masters and guides to us. Water was once again pure and clean. The Earth would once again regain its original innocence.

Something else that occurred to me since the arrival and development of Aqualead was the increased creativity in my life and the desire for self-expression through the arts. While I lived in Belgrano, Buenos Aries, I was surprised by the sudden desire to learn to play the violin and the tin whistle; I found music teachers and soon began playing both musical instruments, in traditional Celtic music. I also began drawing, sketching and later took painting; I also started knitting again, a skill I had abandoned since childhood. It seemed I needed some creative outlets for the energy of Aqualead to express itself. I felt, with the appearance of Aqualead in my life, that the energy was having me re-examine and revive all these artistic venues I had thought buried and lost forever. It is interesting that these old skills I had abandoned decades ago were brought forth by the energy, and were now a central part of my life and even a field of study for me. Once back in Canada, I joined a music school where I still play and practise the violin, and I also went to an art school and learned to paint with acrylics. I also began playing other musical instruments, such as the guitar and the flute.

iii. The road that never ends

Once a person completes the third level and becomes an Aqualead Master, this does not mark the end of their journey. On the contrary, it's only the beginning. Being an Aqualead Master is something that continues to grow on a person perpetually. The energy accompanies you every day in your life, and the guidance and support one receives from it is continuous. As far as I am concerned, not one day goes by when I do not send or use at least one of the symbols. It seems the advanced level of Aqualead steers you into another way of life, where the concept of time no longer applies.

The enhanced intuition from the Aqualead attunements also makes us far more sensitive and perceptive towards others. Any lies, deception or dissimulation is quickly detected, and this makes it difficult to sustain relationships with those who are not honest or in tune with their true inner self. I also found it more difficult to be in places where the energy is either very dense, heavy or negative. In these instances, I found myself using Aqualead all the time to counteract and release the negativity. The feeling of protection and support is amazing from having such an energy around. Whether it is at home, work or school, this energy constantly works, and also acts on others around us. It is a win-win situation. Because the energy is so environmental, I found it made me much more sensitive to issues surrounding the use of harmful chemicals, and animal welfare. I have been much more drawn to growing my own fruits and vegetables in the garden, avoiding herbicides and pesticides, buying organic foods and avoiding brand names that test their products on animals. A huge sense of commitment towards the Earth has developed in me, and I find that the energy of Aqualead is still teaching me on this path.

As an Aqualead Master, I feel more than ever that I am still a student of this modality. The more I teach, the more I learn from others. The Aqualead students also have indirectly served me as valuable teachers and guides, often sharing with me in the class experiences and ideas that I had never heard of myself. My guides, the elementals that accompany me, also have taught me a great deal. And I do feel that this path I was placed on will go ever onward. The changes produced by Aqualead's presence always serve as a reminder of this blessing. This evolution Aqualead is bringing forth in this world starts with those who first learn this energy, and begin practising and sending it. I feel this evolution in me, as I envision a future that may become the course of things now altered. There is a possibility of the world evolving to a simpler, greener way of life, with less dependency on machines and more so on water and trees. It also creates the possibility for the increase in alternative sources of energy instead of fossil fuels, such as cars running on water (which already exist), or more electric cars; as well as in the development of solar and wind power.

These are all simple changes to make, and these changes are already visible. However, there is still a need for more adaptation, and soon. I am not convinced this planet can afford to wait another sixty years continuing on this path, until humanity and its leaders finally change their ways. These changes and developments must happen much more quickly. These modifications will take time to occur; however, the sooner, the better. There is an urgent need for a change in sources of energy, and other alternatives need to be explored. I am hoping that Aqualead's colourful and creative energy will help bring on more innovation and transformation in that respect. Perhaps this would explain Aqualead's crucial timing in entering this world. I feel that this energy has arrived here at the very last minute; and that this arrival is greatly welcome, not only by me but also by others everywhere else in the world.

CHAPTER VI

SPIRITUAL GROWTH AND FURTHER PRACTICES

i. About the Unicorn symbols

These six symbols are an opportunity for Masters to advance their skills and increase their range of practice. These symbols do not constitute a fourth level in the Aqualead Program. In fact, they are not really a part of the Aqualead Program in itself, nor are they considered Aqualead energy. They are an addition to the program, which is optional for the Masters. These symbols have a relation to one of the Aqualead Master symbols, because of the high frequencies of light they harbour. They are tools that can be combined with the Aqualead symbols, which can greatly enhance the effect of a healing session. They provide a deeper healing effect at the emotional level, as they go more in detail in the range of human emotions related to different situations and traumas. The energy of Aqualead in itself can provide emotional healing, as well as physical and mental; however, the additional healing brought on by the Unicorn symbols goes much further in dealing with personal crisis and emotional issues surrounding relationships.

The Unicorn symbols can be very useful in dealing with victims of physical, psychological violence and sexual abuse. These energies go deep into a person's heart and mind, and allow releasing these emotions, bringing them in full view, so the person can observe and re-examine those feelings as they gently dissolve. When people think about Unicorns, we think of these fairy-tale like creatures commonly appearing in children's books. But in reality these beings are much different from the usual association with children's fiction. These are beings of Light with incredible healing abilities. And now, these abilities are shared with us in this world, in order to put them to use for the benefit of others. These symbols can be applied to people of all ages, and can be used for a wide array of emotional-related issues, such as guilt, shame, grief, depression, sleep disorders, anger, fear and the aftermath of physical and sexual assaults. Family-related issues, genetically transmitted problems and unwanted patterns can also be dealt with through one of the symbols.

The Aqualead Masters can also use the Unicorn symbols for self-healing. These constitute a wonderful healing tool for those who have them, and some Masters use these symbols only for healing themselves. It is also a step forward beyond the Aqualead Master level which is well-worth exploring. Aqualead Masters do not require receiving any further attunements in order to learn and use these symbols.

ii. About Queldon

Queldon is a second healing modality that I have channelled on March 31st, 2010, in Buenos Aires. This other new modality came to me from the same source where Aqualead came from; however, there was *no angel* present during its channelling process. This energy was sent to me directly from one of my masters. This energy is *not* Aqualead; it has a different purpose and mission altogether, but still works well in synchronicity with the purpose of Aqualead. Queldon is only practised on human beings; its role is to clear the mind and heart of any blockages, thinking patterns and ideas that may block higher levels of consciousness and hinder human growth. Queldon is here in order to accelerate the evolution process in humanity itself, by releasing these limiting beliefs, addictions and dependencies, in a powerful way. This is an elemental energy, and its form of practice differs greatly from Aqualead. First of all, in Queldon there are no symbols; the obvious reason for this is that no symbols were given to me at all during this channelling process. Also, this energy can only be sent to human beings, one person at a time. The session, unlike Aqualead, does not entail applying the hands over a person; the technique is altogether different.

But what makes Queldon so special is its incredible power, and the rapid shifting of dimensions it brings in its immediate surroundings. The vibration of Queldon is so elevated, it took me a year in order to fully understand it and begin using it. I only taught my first Queldon student on February 24th, 2011, in Buenos Aires, who was Andrés. I later shared Queldon with more friends and Aqualead Masters, such as Marian and Lupe in Martinez, as well as Roberto, Claudia and Claudio in the city of Buenos Aires. This energy likes to stand alone; it is not practised with crystals, or any other healing modalities or symbols. There is very little written information concerning this modality, for it is the energy itself which acts as a master. This energy has an intense presence, almost like a sentient being. And this presence is felt in a Queldon session, and continuously when a person is attuned to it. This energy, I believe, will help heal many negative attachments that hold back humanity in its progression, such as greed, selfishness, the urge to control others and the lust for money.

Being an elemental energy, Queldon, by removing these blockages and barriers, helps remind us of the importance of remembering who we are and where we came from. Queldon transports our consciousness to a higher, more enlightened state, and shifts our awareness towards guarding and protecting the planet. Queldon is therefore considered a more advanced form of healing than Aqualead. It is centred on heightening human consciousness and clearing the path for a more detached way of thinking. It addresses these human patterns and habits, and our tendency to take things for granted without any thought or questioning. And very often, dealing with these patterns means going back into our past history, in order to find their source.

Such an abstract healing modality, with a very high vibration energy such as Queldon, has brought on a new challenge to the Aqualead healers, for those who were up to this challenge. In order to be able to learn Queldon, one must have a minimum of Aqualead level II, and wait a minimum of six months before learning and using this energy. This delay is necessary, in order for the energies from the second attunement of Aqualead to settle in the person and be solidly anchored. Also, it allows time for the person to ascertain whether they really want to learn and practise Queldon. This energy is not for everyone to learn. One must be ready and prepared, in order to receive a Queldon attunement. The energy is very intense, in ways that would be difficult to describe to most people. For this reason, it is better for aspiring Queldon students to try a session in person or remotely, in order to get a feel of the energy beforehand. There are two levels of Queldon: practitioner and Master. In essence, the Master level of Queldon exists in order for the modality to perpetuate itself and spread. Queldon Masters do not have any more additional skills than the practitioners, only the ability to teach and give the attunements. Despite the fact that Queldon is a modality that is taught, there are far fewer people in the world practising Queldon than Aqualead. After departing from Argentina in June 2011, I taught Queldon to only a few people here in Canada the following year, and later in Iceland, in June 2013. On June 28th, 2013, there were only 81 Queldon Masters in the world; 70 were in Argentina, five were in Canada and six in Iceland.

While still living in Buenos Aires, I travelled to Rosario, Santa Fé, and to Capilla del Monte in order to teach both levels of Queldon, in June 2011. Our friend Liliana was among the very first Queldon Masters initiated in Rosario, and is still teaching today. Claudio started many Queldon lineages in Buenos Aires, as well as initiating the very first Queldon

Master from Cordoba City. This modality is only practised and taught to adults. Even though Queldon is a separate modality, it is considered affiliated with the Aqualead Program, due to the fact that the second level of Aqualead is a prerequisite to learning Queldon. However, this marvellous and impressive energy is still considered a completely separate entity on its own.

I have added below a checklist for Aqualead practitioners aspiring to learn Queldon. I hope this checklist proves to be useful and helpful, and shows the importance of preparation, and making a conscious decision before learning this modality. I've also included below some advice to Queldon Masters, before they teach a class.

Advice for Aqualead students in order to help them prepare for Queldon:

- Practise and study Aqualead level II.
- Send distant healing.
- Give yourself an Aqualead session, focusing on the heart.
- Meditate, with or without Aqualead symbols.
- Try a Queldon session, or receiving a distant Queldon session at least once.
- Observe your own energy, as well as others'.
- Be mindful of your thoughts and intentions.
- Drink water and eat lightly.

Advice for Queldon Masters before teaching:

- Make sure the student has had Aqualead level II for at least six months.
- Practice the Queldon self-healing session.
- Ask yourself if the student is ready to receive a Queldon attunement.
- Observe the student's energy.
- Project the intention in the Queldon class that the attunement may serve the highest good of all.
- In order to learn the Master level, the Queldon practitioner must wait a minimum of two months.

iii. Working with crystals

There is a strong affinity between Aqualead and crystals. Aqualead is a high vibration of energy which brings us back to the Earth, and crystals come from the Earth; gemstones are therefore a very useful and helpful tool in energy healing. And in the practise of Aqualead, the use of crystals is constant, not to say at times, essential. Crystals can be used in many ways, such as enhancing the effect of a certain energy, directing or amplifying energy. They can also create a protective space for healing work, transmute lower vibrations, ground and cleanse other stones. Typically, crystals are used in healing work by placing the stone over a person's *chakra*. Also, *elixirs* can be made by leaving a certain crystal in water for several hours; the healing property of the crystal is then absorbed into the water, which is then used for healing. Crystals can also be charged with a certain healing energy and by direct exposure to the sun or the full moon; in that sense, gemstones can be considered *natural batteries*. They have the amazing ability of containing and retaining energy.

In the midst of this vast array of uses crystals possess, they are mainly used in Aqualead to send energy at a distance over a prolonged period of time. There is also a crystal attributed to each one of the symbols, which healers may opt to use in their energy healing work. Clear quartz crystals are natural conductors of energy, and they are most frequently used in energy healing. They conduct, direct, amplify and purify energy, and when placed in a circle or grid, can create a protective energy space. Also, the crystals can easily be programmed to send energy remotely at a distance. Some of the stones that I like to use in my energy work include amethyst, which is one of my favourite crystals. This violet gemstone has the ability to transmute lower negative energies and is highly protective during intensive energy work. It also carries a very spiritual energy vibration, and creates a favourable vibration for sleep and meditation. Another stone I enjoy using is rose quartz. This lovely pink crystal attracts love, romance and heals the heart and emotions. It is excellent to use in difficult times of turmoil and crisis. It is perfect to use in distant healing, for it sends loving and forgiving vibes to the situation, or persons involved. I find rose quartz also makes a great crystal for children.

Citrine is a positive, happy stone that eliminates sadness and grief and brings confidence and core strength. Carnelian is great for grounding and dealing with anger, frustration and resentment. Each crystal carries its own healing property, and when a healer of any discipline incorporates these stones in their practice, the benefits are multiplied tenfold. Using crystals is my most common method of sending energy when I'm at home. Aqualead works especially well with crystals; also, the stones seem to fit in perfectly in the natural setting Aqualead creates. I always love showing crystals to new Aqualead students and I always allow people to hold them in their hand, so they can feel the vibration of the stone. I am always surprised at the amount of people, even those who do healing work, who are not familiar with crystals. I find that a minimal amount of knowledge of crystals is a *must*, not only for energy healers and holistic practitioners, but also for the general public. Even without practising an energy healing modality, using the crystals alone is highly beneficial to everyone, and would save many people a huge amount of stress and other health-related issues.

I personally never leave home without some of my crystals. At home, at work or in music school, I am constantly surrounded by gemstones. After working with crystals for so long, I often feel that these minerals actually possess a life and a will of their own. And at some time in their life, a person may attract a certain crystal, and later the crystal may leave that person once their mission is fulfilled. Crystals always fascinate people who have never seen them before. And I take great pleasure in introducing crystals to people everywhere; and very often when I show them a crystal, I get the initial question: *what's that?* This indicates to me the need to expose society more to healing stones. They are the ambassadors of the Earth. Learning to harness the energy of the stones means commuting with the planet itself, from beneath its surface.

Even ordinary rocks or boulders in a forest are the object of fascination to me. Rocks carry within them an element of strength and eternity. Minerals carry the history of the Earth and the wisdom of nature. They also resonate well with nature beings and elementals, who all resonate with them. Another important role crystals play is that of grounding. They help us maintain our connection to the ground and Earth, and thus prevent us from feeling *spaced out*, during and after performing meditation or any kind of spiritual or energy work.

iv. Additional tools: Meditation, self-healing, using essential oils, music and chanting

In this section I discuss additional tools that Aqualead Masters have used and still apply in their practice. This can also be useful to those who are inexperienced in healing work or are curious to know more about them. I have added all these techniques that I have experimented with, working with other Aqualead Masters while I was living in Argentina.

The experience proved to be most helpful, and enlightening; I still use most of these on a daily basis.

Meditation

I find meditation the essential and most fundamental form of spiritual practice. It is a great exercise for everyone and very easy to do. The Aqualead Program includes meditation in all levels of Aqualead. From the first class, the student is introduced to a meditation. Meditating, I found, was most helpful for all of us, in terms of integrating the energy, getting better acquainted with the symbols and simply allowing our energy to flow with the added new energy of Aqualead.

Self-healing

Throughout all the levels of Aqualead, students are encouraged to practice the self-healing session. In class, it is often this form of healing practice that I give the students to do. Practising in class is most important for the students so they realize they can do it, and also get hands-on experience working with the energy. It is a great confidence builder for beginners and a great healing tool for experienced practitioners and Masters. I still give myself Aqualead healing sessions all the time when needed. It's a part of our daily maintenance. It helps keep our energy channels clear, and keeps our energy and emotions in a centred, balanced state.

Using essential oils

I am by all means not an expert in the field of aromatherapy. However, an essential oil was later attributed by my guides to each of the Aqualead symbols, and this proved to be greatly beneficial as well. I have been using oils all the time, my favourites being tea tree and lavender oils. Simply inhaling the aroma of the oil has a therapeutic property in itself. One or two drops of essential oils can also be added to a glass of water, in order to ingest the healing benefits. These oils are easily absorbed through the skin, and make great massage oils. I always keep lavender oil around the house and find myself, in moments of fatigue and weariness, rubbing the oil on my hands and on my face. The relaxing, soothing effect is almost instant.

Incense is another one of my weak spots. Even though incense is burned and is not applied to the skin, there is nothing like the aroma of a burning incense stick or cone, and the sight of a wisp of smoke streaming upward into the room. The fragrance seems to have a definite healing effect and a cleansing presence wherever it is burnt. My favourite incenses are sandalwood, *Palo Santo* (in natural wood form) and rose.

Music and chanting

As a trained *Kundalini yoga* teacher, I was always taught and made aware of the importance of sound in meditation and healing. Sound is a great carrier for energy vibrations. Either through music, signing or chanting, sound has a powerful healing effect, depending on the tonality and pitch of the note. Each one of our chakras has its own vibration, from the lowest chakra to the highest. If translated into music, we can match these vibrations from the lowest note at the root (lowest) chakra, to the highest note at the crown (highest) chakra. Sound therapy is therefore a valuable and very interesting method of healing.

Instruments that are commonly used to produce these healing sounds are signing bowls, bells, gongs and other Tibetan instruments. Drumming also has a powerful effect and is used in shamanic healing and ceremonies. I had the opportunity to meditate and practise Aqualead energy with groups of practitioners and Masters, while some were using different singing bowls in the room. The effect was powerful. Needless to say, other musical instruments will also have a therapeutic effect. Music played with guitars, drums, violin and song also moves the soul, and blends very well with the practice of Aqualead. In a gathering with other Aqualead Masters in 2011, we chanted the names of some of the Aqualead symbols in the form of mantras. Each syllable of the name was chanted slowly and held for a long time, and I found that carried the sound in a most interesting way.

v. A journey into consciousness

Healing with Aqualead energy proved to be an adventure, not only in the environment with the elements of nature but also to the universe within. It has made many people practise a greater level of detachment to material things and adopt a simpler way of doing things. I have learned through Aqualead that *less is more.* Instead of acquiring material objects and aiming for more material wealth, I valued the elements of nature, the food I ate and every glass of water with gratitude. One thing was appreciated at a time, as I became more grateful to any little thing that came to me. In fact, by adopting this attitude, I came to attract much more than I could ever expect, by learning to let go and eliminating cumbersome clutter from my life.

This proved to be a valuable exercise both in humility and in the art of living from one day to the next despite busy schedules, and living in a busy metropolitan city. Somehow, with the presence of Aqualead, I managed to create an oasis of nature around me with simple things such as plants, crystals, meditating with Aqualead, music, crafts and sketching drawings. I had my own refuge and as I connected more with the Fairy world, I soon realized that it was not necessary to retreat to a forest hundreds of kilometres away in order to encounter elementals. They appeared, tiny, among the leaves of my plants. I could see them in the tall trees alongside the streets of Buenos Aires, at night. I saw that they were there among us and that the trees, parks and gardens in cities were still a part of their range of dwelling.

When I was in my tiny living room in my apartment in Buenos Aires, I would feel the presence of the two same Elves standing behind me, against the wall. The elementals could communicate with me and shared some of their knowledge with me. I would ask them some questions and they would patiently answer me, in thought. There were others appearing as small specks of light, hovering peacefully over the cushions I had on the floor. I could also spot little sparks of light among the leaves of my plants, by the window. This inner retreat with the elementals' presence provided me with an inner journey that I followed, fearlessly and without hesitation. This is a path that I do not regret. As much as I never thought I could connect with Gnomes and Elves with such ease, I understand that this was meant to be for me, and I would not change this part of me for anything in the world. My world is in fact intertwined with their world. We are one.

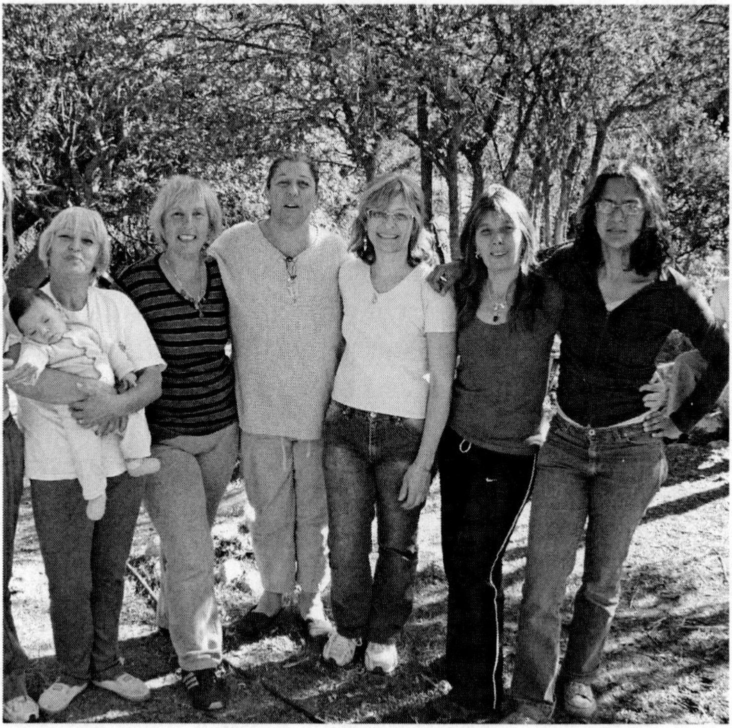

7. *Refugio Paso a Luz*, in Quebrada de Luna, in the province of Córdoba, in November 2009. This was my first time teaching Aqualead to a group of 17 students, in the centre of Argentina. In this picture are the very first Aqualead Masters of Rosario, Santa Fé.

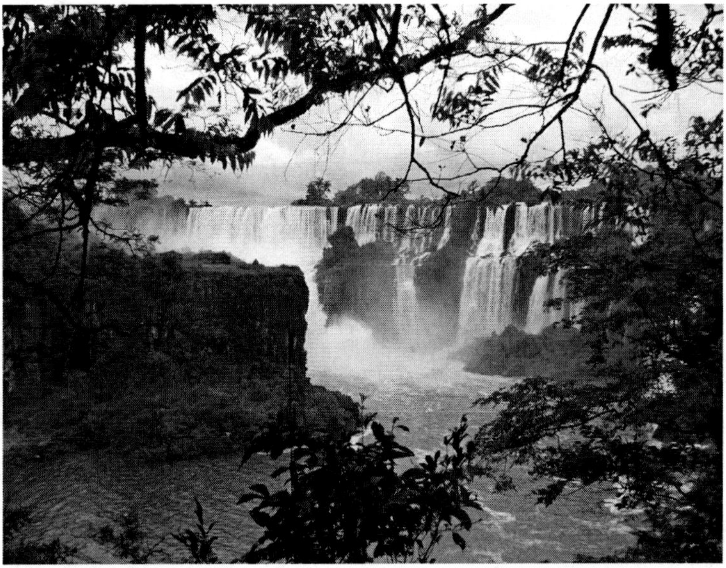

8. Iguazu Falls, in Iguazu National Park in January 2010, in the province of Misiones, Argentina. Three times the size of Niagara Falls, this huge reservoir of water on the Brazilian border was receptive to Aqualead energy.

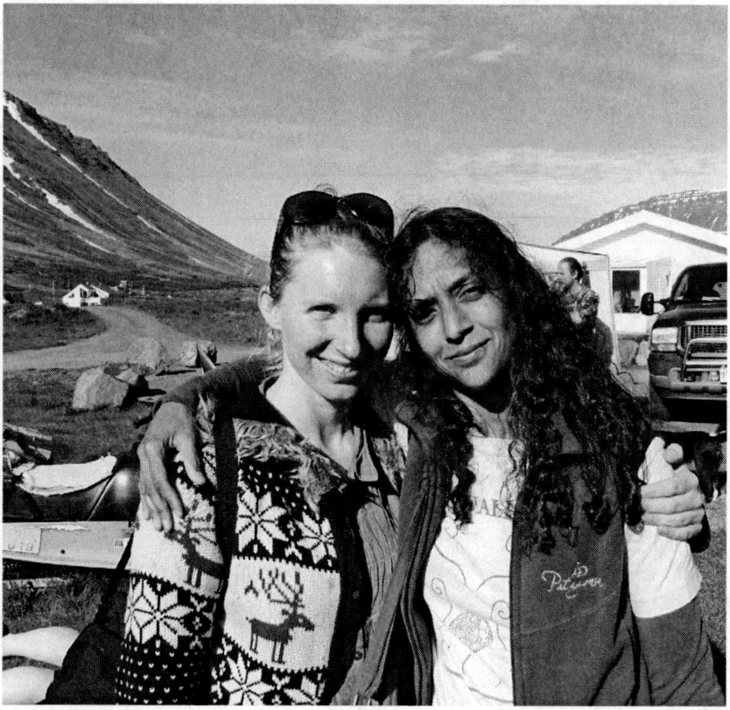

9. My good friend and Aqualead Master Maria Shanko, in Iceland.

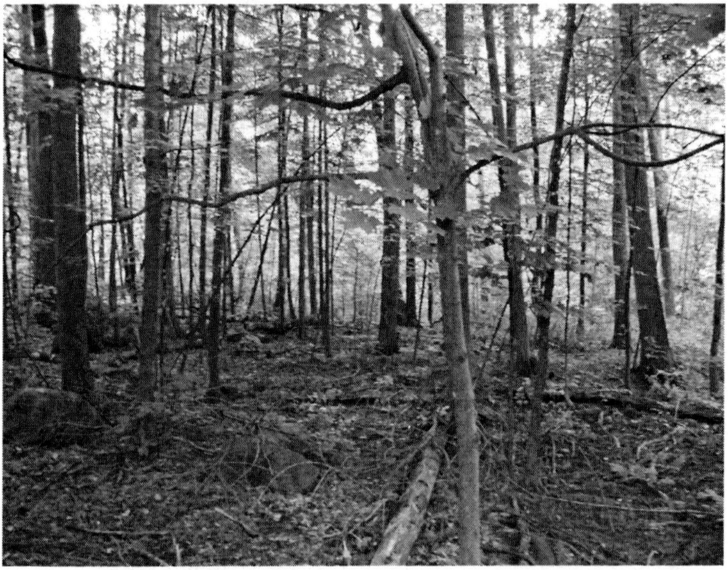

10. Back home, Aqualead blends in perfectly with the woods and rivers of Canada, such as these maple trees in Gatineau Park.

11. There is no place like the garden, especially in the splendour of autumn, in October.

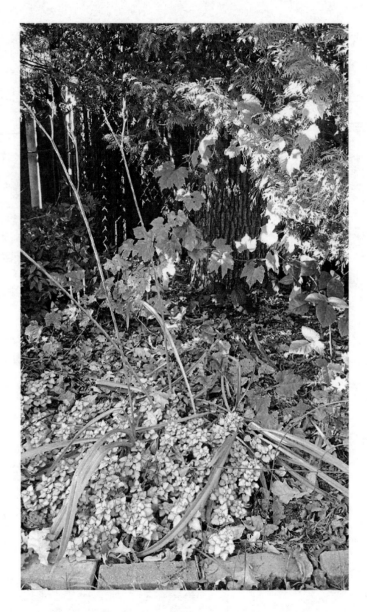

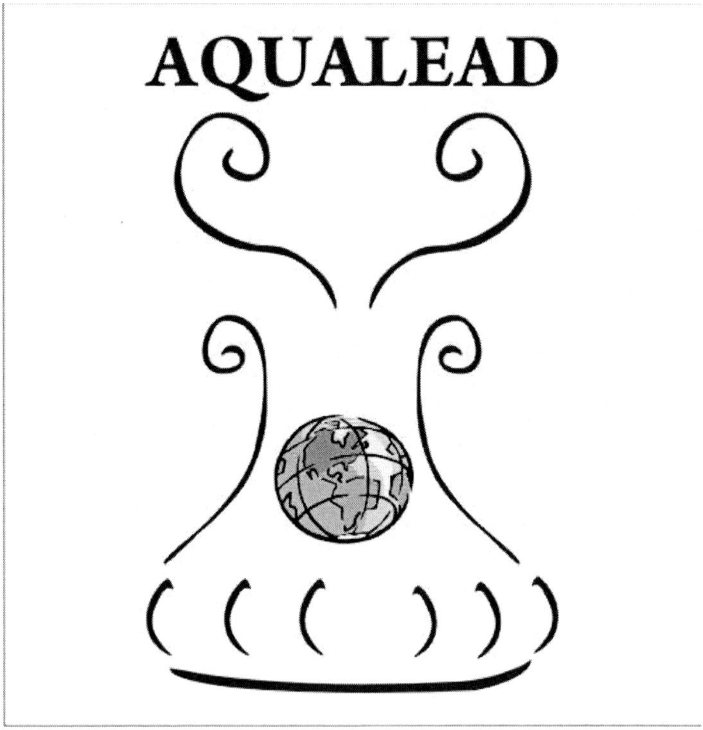

12. The official Aqualead logo, which was produced in Buenos Aires, Argentina in 2009.

PART III

THE RETURN TO NATURE

CHAPTER VII

THE IMPORTANCE OF ELEMENTAL BEINGS

i. Connecting to the Elven realm

Even though I feel them with me all the time, I sometimes get a reminder of the Elves' presence around me. I begin seeing a tiny speck of light in the shadow or in the dark, similar to a spark: it appears and disappears instantly. There is no other lighting in the room at the time, and the manner in which they appear and disappear reminds me of the fireflies I saw when I was younger in my back yard, flickering among the trees. The sight of fireflies always filled me with wonder, as they appeared as Fairies, gracefully passing through the garden among the trees, with their bodies glowing with a clear, bright light in the summer darkness.

The Elves give me that same magical feeling when I know they are near. They also remind me of the importance of working with them, paying attention to their wisdom, focusing our efforts on protecting nature and showing respect towards all its creatures. The elementals are beings of Light, which are equivalent to angels. The main difference is that elementals do not live among humans, and serve a different purpose. These beings specifically dwell in natural habitats, or in any place where the elements of nature exist. Their purpose is to protect and defend nature, especially the trees. Many elementals also defend animals, or focus on protecting a certain part of a natural habitat. Some live in water and in the oceans, and will focus on protecting whales, dolphins and other marine animals.

Elemental beings have great power over the elements of nature, which are for the most part underestimated. They are beings of a higher dimensional space than our own, while being in the same time frame; their energy vibration is therefore of a much higher frequency than that of humans. They are able to shift air currents and create wind gusts; they can also move water and create storms and rough seas. These are phenomenon that would perhaps not be explainable or credible through science. Many sceptics would be quick to refute the idea that elementals beings are responsible for many of the Earth's movements. However, this is what I have observed. Some elemental beings, especially Elves, have great powers and a higher intelligence which are unknown and unseen by the human world.

Elemental beings come in many different shapes and sizes, and go beyond what we may imagine of their realm. The elementals I have spotted may appear very different from one another. Also, most elementals have shape shifting abilities and may take on different forms; for instance, some may take on the appearance of an animal, and may also have a human appearance. However, one can always distinguish the original form of the elemental being, because it will be its most predominant appearance. The Kelpies are an example of this: they are Celtic water horses and generally appear as a dark or white pony along riverbanks, but they may also take a human appearance in order to lure wandering travellers near the water. Some elementals may take on the appearance of insects such as bees, wasps, butterflies and of certain birds. Certain types of elementals have the strange ability to camouflage themselves into rocks, stones and mountains. Some may appear larger in size, and take on colossal proportions as seen with the Giants. Others may also seem rather unattractive or unsightly, such as Goblins and Trolls. Elementals can also display a frightening appearance, and even be hostile towards humans; nature beings that intimidate humans are usually guardians of a certain place or area, keeping intruders away. This does not necessarily mean that they are evil or associated with negative spiritual entities.

There are also various types of elemental beings, which I will refer to as different *races*. The most common ones are the Fairies; the term *Fairies* refers to a type of elemental being, however, the word *Fairy* has also been used to designate all elemental beings. Other common elemental races known in popular culture and folklore are Gnomes, Elves, Dwarves and Giants. The terms *Gnome*, *Fairy* and *elemental beings* have taken on so many forms and different variations depending on culture, local folklore and language that it is difficult to ascertain which elemental is which, among each country or location. For instance, there are many variations of the household elemental which dwells in human homes, according to tradition. In England they are known as Brownies; in Germany they are the Kobolds, in Slavic folklore they are known as *Domovoy*, and in Scandinavia, the *Tomte*. It is difficult to determine whether these beings are really different races of elementals, or simple variations of a common elemental. However, some have their own characteristics, which define them more as an individual kind of nature being in its own right.

Fairies are usually seen in the leaves of smaller plants and love sitting in flowers. Due to their generally smaller size, they like the shady areas under a leaf; they also enjoy the brushy branches of evergreen trees. In the back yard, I sometimes see them in our cedar hedge, near the house. Many Fairies take on a feminine form; however, Fairies may also appear as male, while others do not have any particular gender. These beings can blend in with the trees or even be a part of a tree; some may have branches or leaves extending from their head or limbs. Fairies are graceful, luminous beings and are widespread in different parts of the world. There is also an association between the Fairies and the elements of air, fire, water and earth. They are deeply rooted to their environment and guard the basic elements of nature by their presence.

Gnomes are also small in size, about three to 18 inches tall, and have a more elderly appearance. They often have beards; they are highly intelligent, crafty and ingenious. They are the hard-working, dedicated fosterers of nature. They are the ones often referred to as the *Little People*. They mainly play a role of caretakers, looking after plants, trees and gardens. They will also care for animals, and help those in distress. Gnomes are found in just about every continent in the world, however, may take on different forms and different names. They can build small houses, furniture, bridges and use carts and wheelbarrows.

The Elves are tall, graceful beings of human size; however, some may be taller. They have prominent powers and have strong healing abilities. Their energy vibration is generally higher than that of other elementals. They have a high intelligence and have a higher level of wisdom and understanding than other elemental beings. They sing and love music and sometimes their voices can be heard echoing in the woods; they also have great crafting abilities and can make various things, such as musical instruments, clothing and housing structures. Elves are practically invisible in the woods, as well as their homes.

Dwarves have a short, stout stature and live mainly underground and underneath mountains. They have a strong affinity for rocks and stones. They have great physical strength and endurance, and can dig tunnels and chambers underground for many years. They live in closely-knit family groups, and work with a combination of the elements of fire and earth. They are great metal smiths.

Giants are magnificent, large elemental beings that play a unique role in the world. They are the guardians and keepers of the Earth's history. Very connected to rocks and stones, Giants are also shape-shifters and can mould themselves into a mountain or hillside. They have great longevity, and their size can range from nine feet tall to hundreds of feet. Many can cause earthquakes and are involved in the cycles of mountains and volcanoes. Other known races of elemental beings are Pixies, Leprechauns and Mermaids.

Elemental beings are physical living beings, however some present similar characteristics to spiritual entities. The term *nature spirits* is more than likely associated with their higher intelligence and their inherent invisibility. Elemental beings are invisible and imperceptible to the majority of people, which makes them difficult to discuss, or describe in a concrete way. There have been many sightings of elemental beings worldwide, but one requires a higher, more intuitive perception in order to be able to consciously see them. The concept of nature beings or elementals creates a clash with the fast-paced urban noise of the modern world. Elementals have a very long life span, such as hundreds of years while some may be immortal; each type of elemental has its own energy vibration, and some who have a denser energy vibration may have more definite or shorter life spans. Immortal elementals would be those more closely related to higher vibrations of light. They have powers that are difficult to understand to us; however, these abilities are real.

Despite human developments and urbanization, elementals will always send us a sign of their presence, and that the invisible forces of nature are not yet extinct. There is a certain advanced race of elemental beings living underground; they once dwelled on the surface of the Earth, and were forced to retreat beneath the surface when the human race began to proliferate. This ancient race of beings is called *the Sidhe*, and is known as the *Good People* in Ireland. They are able to communicate with us and remind us of their presence.

ii. Surrounded by the Fairy world

Despite scepticism, the presence of elementals has been recorded by human mortals for centuries. In many different cultures, tradition and mythologies, elementals have appeared in one form or another. Human culture is embedded with the presence of elementals, without people actually noticing. The *Green Man* mythology is well-known, as well as the tradition of *Santa Claus* and the Christmas Elf. The *Nymphs*, which are female nature deities, are deeply embedded in Greek mythology. Fairy tales from the Brothers Grimm, Hans Christian Andersen and the rich Icelandic and Scandinavian folklores are filled with tales of Gnomes, Fairies and Elves. Throughout the world, the Nature People seem to have made their mark, and have inspired humanity with their grace for centuries, as early as Shakespeare's *A Midsummer Night's Dream*. In this classic play, Oberon is the king of Fairies and Elves, who live in a forest. Belief in elemental beings is closely intertwined with ancient Celtic beliefs, paganism and aboriginal ways of life. It seems to stem from a way of life which implies honouring the forces of nature and being attentive to its cues and signals. It also implies a holistic view of the world and of nature, instead of seeing the natural world as a threat, or something which needs to be contained or controlled.

It seems as though the elementals still surround us continuously, despite humanity's impression of having dominion over the Earth. For millions of years, there have been elemental beings on Earth, while humans live relatively brief lifetimes in the world, thinking they are alone. Meanwhile these elementals are probably hundreds of years old, and are still here among us. Are they waiting for the next drastic change? Do they know anything about the fate and future of humanity? Only they would know the answer. Since the fabric of the planet is of a mineral origin, many elementals live underground and underneath the mountains. They are connected to all the crystals in the Earth, and have been holding the Earth's history for millions of years.

The presence of elemental beings is reminding humanity that we are not alone, even though we may think we are. Humans are not the only intelligent race on Earth, and there is a greater need for awareness of our actions, which have consequences for the lives of others. The elemental beings remind us that humanity is not an isolated island on this planet, nor can we claim any power over it. The Earth owns us, and we are only a part of this ancient web of life. Elemental beings are among us and surround us in order to add a different light in the world and keep us connected to the magical worlds they dwell in. There are many ways to connect to the elemental beings' energies and work with them in protecting and caring for nature. Using Aqualead is most useful in achieving this.

iii. Aqualead and the elemental realm

There is a great affinity between the work of Aqualead practitioners and Masters, and the elemental world. Both have the same level of awareness towards the planet's situation, and are willing and ready to act in order to deal with these issues. Furthermore, the energies that Aqualead Masters work with are somewhat similar to the elemental's energies. Some of the Aqualead symbols have a magnetic effect on Fairies and will increase their presence and power. The energy is fully supportive to them and enables them to be more visible, stronger and more perceptible to the lower human dimension. The Aqualead symbol used in the second level for plants and agriculture also has a strong affinity with the elemental world and attracts Fairies. It was common to hear accounts of new Aqualead students beginning to see Gnomes on their homes, or spotting Fairies in their gardens and flower beds.

The presence of Aqualead and the work of the Aqualead communities enable elemental beings to work with them as a team effort in order to help rebalance the planet. In exchange, the elementals can also work with the Aqualead practitioners and Masters, in order to achieve a common goal. This makes the healing work on the planet much more effective, interactive and dynamic. Since Aqualead's arrival and the increased awareness of elemental beings, there has been much energy shifting and moving throughout the world. Here, we begin to see two worlds converging, human mortal and elemental, as humans are beginning to reach a higher level of dimension. It makes it much easier to work with the Elven race and other elementals, in order to create a bridge for greater communication and understanding.

It is my hope that Aqualead will help reduce this energy gap between humans and other beings. There is currently a huge clash of energies happening worldwide as the adaptation to a higher dimensional state is achieved. It is a difficult and strenuous adaptation for some: perhaps the energy of Aqualead will also help reconcile and harmonize the huge conflict between human interests and the survival and balancing of ecosystems on Earth. This transformative phase occurring in the world may be greatly enhanced and even exacerbated by this new balance. Sending Aqualead healing remotely at a distance implies directly working with the elemental's energies and joining our efforts with theirs. It also acknowledges their presence, as we put the essence and magic of nature back to where it belongs; this is not meant to disempower the human race but only to balance the excessive use of force by humanity in establishing their place in the world. The natural world should not be compromised in this equation, and this is where the balancing needs to occur.

CHAPTER VIII

RELATIONSHIPS WITH ANIMALS

i. Bridging the gap

The topic of healing animals in the scope of Aqualead tends to be a sensitive subject. To most people, healing animals is focused on household cats and dogs, and the relationships they have with their human masters. In Aqualead, however, healing animals goes farther and deeper than this. As a modality centred on defending the Earth and healing the environment, the energy has brought up certain truths and issues concerning the treatment of animals, which are not pleasant to see. As much as Aqualead favours a closer connection to animals, communicating and working with animals, the energy also has exposed the realities surrounding the astronomical amount of animal cruelty intertwined within human societies. This is where the energy of Aqualead is pushing the limits of human understanding and acknowledging that certain things *must change* in human habits, in order for peace and balance on Earth to be established. The pace of this transformation process depends on how much people are willing to change, and how easily they can let go of certain traditions and consumption habits. This is where Aqualead can assist in transforming this situation and transmuting these lower, aggressive energies into more Light and compassion.

In order to change a situation, the *energy* of it most likely needs to be changed to bring a more positive outcome. It may seem difficult to understand how energy healing work can alter the course of events, yet it *does*. In energy healing everything counts, and any healing energy sent accumulates and builds up, until results begin to show. The light has many different ways of entering the world in order for it to do its work. It is therefore difficult to predict how these changes may occur, and the progression or time frame in which this may happen. This is why energy healing is a subject that is so difficult to grasp by many, as these subtle energies work in ways beyond the healer's control. Like other healing energies, Aqualead energy is *intelligent* and may act in ways beyond the knowledge and understanding of the healer who sends it. In the scope of healing animals and protecting them from harm, this same concept applies.

At the first level of Aqualead, the student is initiated to the *animal communication* symbol. It is not coincidental that this symbol was placed in the first level of Aqualead, at the beginner level. It seems that connecting with animals and developing empathy for them is just as fundamental as doing the energy work on water and healing green spaces. The energy of this symbol does not work by healing water, but rather through communication and the consciousness of animals. This symbol is used to enhance communication with the animals, and enhance our ability to connect to their thoughts and feel their emotional states. The introduction of this symbol to the Aqualead Program greatly enhanced our sensitivity to the animal kingdom and I had received myriad messages about animals, and the need to heed their distress calls of suffering. As one's consciousness expands, there is a greater understanding and sensitivity towards the treatment of other creatures, and the desire to return animals held captive to freedom. This awareness in Aqualead is inherent and fundamental.

In Aqualead the understanding of the freedom of animals and their right to live is automatic. The understanding that animals have basic rights is commonly acknowledged; it is a simple step towards showing respect to other living creatures. This respect will extend further when we realize that we are in fact not a superior species to others, and must leave room for other ecosystems and habitats to thrive. If we are to survive as a species, we must learn to modify and change our habits so they do not hinder or compromise other species' right to live in a state of complete freedom. We must reflect on certain issues, such as our model of *animal agriculture*, which entails the genetic manipulation, raising and slaughter of billions of animals. We need to re-examine these unnecessary practices, and the extent of the environmental damage, animal cruelty and the huge waste of food and water it creates. This is where a heightened awareness can shed some light on these issues and bring a better outcome for all living creatures on Earth.

Slaughterhouses create an endless chain of misery and suffering to innocent animals. The healing energy work may on one side enhance the compassion of humans, and also help protect these animals and hopefully bring them freedom from this type of treatment. And as long as there are animals that are being held captive and experimented on, or exploited in zoos, circuses and aquariums, it will be very difficult for the human race to evolve and transcend this level of selfishness. The healing needs to take place from the angle of breaking patterns, which hinder evolution. And this is the most difficult barrier and obstacle to break, for the sake and love of the animals of the Earth. I know that many people become defensive and angry when confronted with those realities. Most people have a pet in their home and at the same time support the most cruel and destructive industries in the world. This is a common contradiction that creates an emotional situation when brought up to the light. And the changes begin from within society, with the consumers.

The energy of Aqualead remains strongly centred around the issue of animals and their welfare. Animals are the children of the Earth and remain the custodians of the planet. As early as the first level, this awareness and consciousness about animals and the need to respect them is emphasised to the students. However, healing and working with animals' issues is not always a pleasant type of work. One must see the immense suffering of these animals, which unfortunately are used and consumed through these different industries as mere objects. This is a huge issue that Aqualead is releasing and bringing out into the open for all to see. Healing the

Earth and including the animals in the equation does not limit itself to showing a basketsful of kittens. And beyond the relationships people maintain with their household dogs and cats, the awareness or sensitivity often ends there. This is where a higher sense of justice is in the process of establishing itself, and where the light needs to enter the most, for the sake and survival of wildlife and other unfortunate animals.

ii. Balancing the ecosystems

Aqualead is a healing energy but also has a strong protective aspect to it. This is why we send so much Aqualead to the endangered species; for instance, to these animals who are unfortunately being poached for their ivory. In this case, the focus of the healing should also be sent to those who generate a demand for this cruel trade. The extent of Aqualead's protection can also be directed at all the whales and dolphins that are being unnecessarily hunted. All these animal species that are under attack by humans will benefit from the energy, which is hopefully helping protect them from extinction. The energy can also help raise awareness on the fragility of these ecosystems the human race is constantly attacking and plundering. Any unbalance in nature and its ecosystems can be dealt with by Aqualead, but some time may be required until the results begin to show, especially on a planetary scale. As a part of balancing the Earth, ecosystems are an essential part of the environment as they are the movement of life and water on this planet.

Any imbalance in this world regarding animal populations is directly related to human activity. In the oceans this imbalance is largely related to commercial fishing, which has taken on huge and abusive proportions. This fishing done with nets has contributed to the drowning of dolphins, sharks and whales that become ensnared in them. This has destabilized the marine ecosystems, while the commercial killing of sharks for their fins has depleted the oceans even more. This greed and massive overconsumption has led to persistent depletion of life on Earth. And this overconsumption is completely unnecessary and detrimental to a fragile network of living species, which has taken millions of years in order to evolve and thrive. Harmful and toxic chemicals have also contributed to the destruction of pristine marine wildlife, as well as offshore drilling for fossil fuels. I found myself sending huge amounts of Aqualead energy to the oceans; this amount of energy work needs to be done also in group healing, and with the help of crystals. However, I still find Aqualead energy works powerfully in all the oceans, which are the cradle of evolution.

This only shows the necessity of a more focused energy healing that is directed towards the water itself and to the planet in its entirety. Much energy healing needs to be sent; groups healing are most effective in order to deal with these situations. The energy may not stop these occurrences immediately;

however, changing the energy inherent in the situation is a good start. Also, the violence absorbed by the water can also be released, in order to remove this pollution from the water and help the environment return to a more original state of innocence. Any minute effort counts and one should not underestimate the effect a single person may have on the rest of the world.

Aqualead focuses on these issues directly and the more this energy is sent worldwide, the better chances wildlife everywhere can be supported and protected against these human abuses. Aqualead is here to teach us the art of simplicity; and by reducing our overall consumption, *we all gain.* By avoiding certain products that are toxic and harmful to our own bodies, we benefit health wise. By avoiding certain foods which are dangerous to produce for animals and the environment, we gain not only with our own health; we all benefit by sparing the Earth more pollution, climate change and deforestation. Everyone benefits if we eat lower on the food chain and avoid meat and other animal products; this improves our health, our safety and ensures a better hygiene of what we eat. Plants, grains, seeds and nuts offer an equal source of protein to animal muscles and organs; nuts and leafy greens are a great source of calcium instead of cow's milk. Plant-based milks are easily made from soy, almonds, coconut, oats or sunflower seeds and are easy to find in supermarkets; they can also be easily made at home with a blender.

Humans are the only species on Earth to maintain the practice of consuming the milk of another species and making it their own food. Despite having grown up in a background which supports it, I now find this practice peculiar and completely illogical. Adults *do not need* to drink milk: it is especially formulated to provide for the needs of the mother's infant. The milk of a lactating mother is purely destined for its offspring. Mammals produce milk to ensure the protection, nourishment and antibodies *for their own young*, in order to ensure their survival in the early moments of life. That is the natural function of milk; this substance is not destined to become a commodity or source of food for a foreign species, to consume throughout adulthood for pleasure. And this is even more unnatural when this practice is done on a mass industrial scale, where millions of cows are exploited, artificially inseminated and their calves are taken away from them in order to be killed. This bizarre and cruel habit of using another species' milk for human consumption needs to be seriously re-examined and reassessed. We must consider the origins of these products we purchase in supermarkets, *how* they are obtained and their effects on human health; and then ask ourselves: *is this truly worth it?*

Avoiding animal-based foods may be a matter of choice, but by choosing this path of consumption and leaving animals out of the equation, we also choose to honour the Earth and animals in a real and genuine way. By making small changes in our daily habits, we can live on a healthier, more balanced planet where we can breathe cleaner air, and drink pure water that is free of dangerous chemicals. In addition, animals will live free and respected, as we all benefit from living in a more peaceful world. It also gives us the peace of mind of knowing that we are leaving this legacy behind to our children and grandchildren, for many centuries to come.

The practice of hunting has been done for thousands of years by humans in order to survive. Most, if not all, aboriginal cultures have practised hunting for the same reasons throughout the centuries. It is perfectly understandable that aboriginal societies may hunt, especially when living under harsh conditions in order to survive, such as through long winters in the North. Native cultures who hunted before the arrival of the Europeans in America hunted only what they needed with rudimentary weapons, and this practice was done with respect. This did not entail the breeding and abuse of animals on a large scale. Modern society has moved far away from this ancient way of life in harmony with nature. It seems we have all grown desensitized to eating the flesh animals we have never seen alive, or killed ourselves. This distance with animals and the elements has contributed to an imbalance in society, which has led us to take certain commodities for granted. We also have moved far away from the original purpose of hunting, where now the hunting of animals is done as a ruthless sport, where animals are shot at with firearms, and often left injured.

iii. Healing speciesism

Some definitions of the word *speciesism* cited from *thefreedictionary.com* go as follows:

spe·cies·ism (spē′ shē-zĭz′əm, -sē-)

n.

Human intolerance or discrimination on the basis of species, especially as manifested by cruelty to or exploitation of animals.

(The American Heritage Dictionary of the English Language. Houghton Mifflin Company, Fourth Edition, 2000.)

spe′cies·ist′ *adj. & n.*

Here is another definition:
speciesism [□spi: □i: z□□z□m]

n

(Life Sciences & Allied Applications / Environmental Science) a belief of humans that all other species of animals are inferior and may therefore be used for human benefit without regard to the suffering inflicted

[from species + -ism]

speciesist *adj*
(Collins English Dictionary – Complete and Unabridged. HarperCollins Publishers, 1991, 1994, 1998, 2000, 2003.)

This word was first coined by Richard D. Ryder in 1970 during his campaigns against the use of animals in laboratory experiments. The term was later used by Peter Singer in his book *Animal Liberation* published in 1975. This term is hardly ever used in the English vocabulary and is rarely seen or read in books or in common media of communication. This word, however, refers to the *discrimination of other species.* The issues of racial, sexual and religious discrimination and sexism were already exposed and are still in full view. These are problems that are restricted within our own human race. But, when we begin to extend our compassion beyond our own kind, things seem to become more complicated. It is strongly my belief that there is nothing that cannot be transformed, and healed. It is only a matter of time, and concentrating the necessary effort where it is needed.

Aqualead is very helpful in dealing with these philosophical issues surrounding animal rights. Here we enter the realm of ideas and ways of thought, which lead many societies to view animals as inanimate objects without any intelligence, feeling or right to respect. The Aqualead agriculture symbol is great at enhancing this compassion towards animals. When coupled with the animal communication symbol, this can greatly assist people in being more aware of other sentient beings. The transformation symbol is also ideal, because this is an abstract concept that steps out of the realms of nature, water and trees. It can help transform and dissolve old thinking patterns, and clear the way for new ways of thinking and seeing others. Aqualead is a very helpful tool in that sense, and can help us reach out and show more concern towards others. This way the healing reaches those who are truly in need of it, and not only to those who are close to us, as a means of convenience.

We can see a progression in humanity towards a greater level of consciousness and general evolution in the human way of thinking. Many obstacles were overcome and some barriers have been broken. This progress has taken centuries of struggle, and a series of often bloody revolutions and campaigns by activists as a catalyst for social change. The changes have taken place; however, the awakening has occurred slowly, and often at the expense of the lives of human rights activists who stood up to the discrimination and general ignorance. However, a greater challenge is now posed in front of the human race, in terms of pushing the limits even further. This means acknowledging the rights of other non-human species, and accepting that the human race is not the superior one on this planet. This also means realizing that enslaving animals and holding them captive against their will is clearly unacceptable, and a violation of their rights.

This also entails, through the concept of speciesism and the discrimination of animals, the questioning of ownership over another intelligent being. Viewing another species as an expendable specimen in a laboratory would also constitute a violation of these rights. The lives of animals are no less important or inferior to that of humans, and it is then not acceptable to use these beings as laboratory subjects for researching diseases, drugs or cosmetics, for the so-called benefit of mankind. The benefit and safety of these animals, meanwhile, would be ignored, denied and disrespected. It seems easy and convenient to turn a blind eye on this treatment of animals, but this needs to be looked at objectively. The love of animals then reaches out to all creatures, as *all* of these animals held captive in pet shops, circuses, factory farms, research facilities and aquariums worldwide are not forgotten. The energy of Aqualead has already gone to them; no one is forgotten or left behind.

This is the formidable healing task we all have to work with the energy, and help bridge this gap of misunderstanding, and consequently not allow this selfish treatment of animals to be tolerated anymore in this world. However, with more cooperation and participation from everyone, we gather strength in numbers. The more energy work is sent, the more healing can occur, and the more consciousness and sensitivity is raised throughout this process. In the scope of Aqualead training, practitioners and Masters are not required to adopt a vegetarian or vegan diet. However, the energy will often lead people towards this trend, as some people began expressing a feeling of repulsion towards meat, eggs or dairy products.

CHAPTER IX

AMONG THE TREES

i. A shamanic view of the world

Some similarities were drawn between the practice and philosophy of Aqualead and Native American shamanism. *Shamanism* is the practice in which the person may reach a higher level of consciousness and encounter supernatural beings; the shaman may also have access to different energies they can channel, in order to practise rituals, divination and healing. Even though Aqualead is not a religion, it creates a close bond to nature and its elements. It also links one to the elemental beings, who are often mistaken for spiritual entities. Shamans are natural healers and have a constant connection to the spiritual world; however, their spiritual connection is closely intertwined with nature and the animal world. To the aboriginal people, Spirit is everywhere: in trees, rocks, rivers as well as in birds and animals. Aqualead practitioners and Masters are often drawn to shamanic healing and practices, through the closeness they share with the elements of nature. Other practices are also intertwined in both shamanism and Aqualead, such as the use of natural herbs, essences, sound, drumming and chanting. Meditation also seems to be a common-place practice.

Due to the fact that Aqualead supports the rebalancing of nature and of animal life, the energy is supportive to an aboriginal way of life, which works in harmony with the forces of nature. Before the arrival of Europeans to the Americas, Native cultures thrived and flourished freely. They lived in harmony in nature and took only what was needed, however this balance was upset with the arrival of Europeans, where the Native People were completely uprooted from their ancient culture and ways of life. Even today in these surviving cultures, they are a small minority and many are confined to living in Indian reserves. Most of these great civilizations are now a memory of the past in the midst of modern society, within ever-growing urban areas. Much Aqualead energy was sent to the Amazon, in order to help protect the rainforest and the Native People's homes. Along with a group of Aqualead healers mainly located in Argentina, we sent distant healing to this large expanse of rainforest and to those interested in exploiting it. The objective was to protect it and hopefully curb deforestation activities, especially surrounding the *Belo Monte* dam issue in Brazil. The project *Aqualead for the Amazon* was created in 2010 in order to address these conflicts surrounding aboriginal rights and the depletion of the Amazon rainforest. I personally found the transformation symbol most useful in these types of situations. It is my hope that the energy of Aqualead can help assist is reducing these damaging activities, within these complex ecosystems.

Aside from supporting the rights of aboriginals and their way of life, Aqualead is also helping all of us adopt a more natural lifestyle, by acknowledging the world of magic, spirits and the natural forces which surround us. As much as science depicts a world devoid of Spirit or soul, Aqualead is putting the *soul* back into the environment. Through this shamanistic view of the world, Aqualead guides us to see animals as powerful totems, spiritual guides and wise beings, instead of mere objects at our disposal. The energy can also teach us to draw more of our own energy from within ourselves, instead of heavily depending on nature. Perhaps it's time for us to tap into our own personal power, and learn to generate our own energy and support; and eventually have the energy to *give back* to the Earth, in the form of gratitude and positive action. This way, we embrace the magical properties of the wizards.

ii. Conversations with the forests

Trees have always captivated my attention as the tall masters and gentle giants of this planet. They stand as the silent rulers, quietly providing oxygen to the fragile network of life on Earth. Just the thought that our breathable air is mostly due to the presence of trees, fills me with wonder and amazement. This also demonstrates the innate perfection and intelligence found in nature. The trees are basically *our lungs*. As important living beings, they have quickly become the focus of attention and healing work in the practice of Aqualead. They are not only a part of the world; they also occupy a position of power for their height, stature, the shade and shelter they provide and for supplying the Earth with water from their roots and oxygen in the atmosphere. Trees are living creatures that share a consciousness with other surrounding trees. They hold the energy space through their hidden consciousness and intelligence, and their ability to respond to energy.

I remember beginning to send Aqualead energy to the trees, and feeling the tree absorbing the energy, eagerly receptive. I also recall, in some instances, the tree sending energy back to me, reciprocating. Trees have a powerful presence and the ability to communicate. I realize that they receive, relay and send off energies, possibly relaying messages to other trees. I cannot help to think at times that trees are like natural antennas, connecting the Earth to the outward universe. In the second level of Aqualead, I had added a *tree meditation* in order to give students the incentive and opportunity to practise sitting close to a tree and establish a connection to it. In groups, I have noticed trees tending to form a collective energy or group consciousness, and form one gigantic being, like a school of fish or a swarm of flying insects.

A forest is a giant, living, breathing entity. Aqualead energy supports the conservations and preservation of natural habitats, in order to keep them untouched. Energy work can easily be blended in with a hike in the woods or a visit to a local park or ecological reserve. Trees and plants also highly benefit from the presence of crystals. The first healing symbol and the plant symbol at the second level of Aqualead are also very suitable for forests, the countryside and other plants living together in groups.

iii. Gardening and recycling with Aqualead

What greater and more wonderful way of contributing to the environment than to recycle waste. We are seeing some signs of positive changes; for instance, as plastic shopping bags are becoming banned in several countries and locations while reusable cloth shopping bags have been making a comeback instead. Recycling and transformation are a common topic in Aqualead healing, since the energy has a strong transformative effect and is very effective at transmuting lower negative energies. We *all* have something in our lives that needs to be recycled. This recycling is a form of cleansing and clearing emotional and physical clutter. This makes room for newer energies in our lives and inviting the universe to send us new beginnings. As much as the world needs to be cleansed, our immediate surroundings and our past also need the same kind of attention.

There is also a growing trend in reusing objects and waste into innovative and artful new things. It is possible to take a used, finished item and transform it into something else, as opposed to buying new things all the time. An example is painting old tires and reusing them as garden ornaments. Others also have used recycled materials into building and insulating houses. Empty plastic bottles can be cut and made into pots for the garden. Some have cut holes into empty metal cans in order to make them into lanterns. The possibilities are endless; and these alternative uses for recyclable materials may be the solution to recycling, managing waste and obtaining new things by crafting and working on old, unwanted objects. Unwanted things around the house or garage then become homemade works of art, and the product of an ingenious craft. This is a part of the process of creativity and transformation.

Home agriculture has also been on the rise and is expanding. More and more people feel the desire to grow their own produce from home, and even share with neighbours. Home gardening and community agriculture could be the future for many towns and even within bigger city centres. Gardening is an excellent way to put Aqualead energy to use. It is a grounding activity, and links one to the roots of the soil and the plants. It is also a fun activity for kids. By including the energy of Aqualead, in the process of gardening and the planting of trees, entering the garden can become a magical experience, which has been noticed by many. Charging the water used in gardening with Aqualead is also an excellent way to use the energy; it is a great idea to use the environmental symbol in the water before watering the garden and trees.

Planting shrubs, perennials and trees is a fun and creative activity. However, planting in pots is just as rewarding. My favourite herbs are mint, lemon grass, dill weed and lavender. Hardy roses are also a favourite, as well as raspberries, strawberries and currants. Rosemary and peppers are easily grown in pots and offer anyone a chance to put their hands in the garden, even in the tiniest of spaces. It seems as though there is a natural synergy between the energy of Aqualead and the act of planting something in the earth. It also enhances the connection with elementals in the garden, who are never too far away. Home gardening for the kitchen also provides organic foods just outside the door. Lettuces and cherry tomatoes are very easy to grow, and share with others. It's a win-win situation. It seems the energy of Aqualead is encouraging the world to become greener, by adding and creating more plant life and natural green spaces.

The greenery can also be created indoors. The mere presence of houseplants is enough to change the energy inside a house, and create a more natural atmosphere. Houseplants improve the quality of air inside a home or apartment, and absorb lower energies. Many have commented on the effect Aqualead has on a plant which seems to be dying, and was revived almost instantly by simply laying their hands over the plants with the basic healing symbol.

AFTERWORD

The presence and practice of Aqualead in the world already has a huge impact on its surroundings. The use of Aqualead has a multitude of facets, like the surface of a diamond. Healing water is only the beginning of the vast amount of change and consciousness this new energy can bring in our lives, and to the environment. I look back at these past years with gratitude and a bit of nostalgia; the first five years of Aqualead's history marks the beginning of a new era; however, these early years of discovery and change will never return. It seems we have passed an initial critical phase, and now that the healing system is well established, it is clearly time to move forward on this new path laid before us.

This is not an individual path for me: this is everyone's individual path, as well as a path we all share together. As Aqualead continues to grow, we grow. And with every growth spurt, there is a necessary rearrangement, which can bring growing pains, like with the upbringing of a child. As we move forward with this new journey with Aqualead, we continue learning new experiences and ways of being. And this journey could not be accomplished without all those who became involved in this incredible and memorable process.

Today, Aqualead continues to thrive and spread in different parts of the world. However, the progression seems to be slower here in North America. Surely there is reason for this and I do not question this slower activity here in the North. I focus more on sending distant healing and working with crystals; I find myself working more on the environmental and social levels remotely at a distance, with the energy. When students are ready, they contact me to schedule a class date. Some things take longer to achieve, and I respect this element of timing. It seems the modality has finished its initial rapid climb and is now levelling off, to its normal cruising altitude. It seems Aqualead is now firmly anchored and established in the world, and moving on with its own momentum. There was an approximate total of 1, 367 Aqualead Masters worldwide as of November 13th, 2013. The energy seems to know well in advance where it needs to expand, and at what pace; I simply follow the energy's signals, and hope it will continue touching the hearts of many more people worldwide.

The more people know about Aqualead and learn it, the more people can harness this incredible new energy, which is opening new possibilities for a better future. As the number of Aqualead practitioners increases worldwide, more changes can occur throughout the world. Then, the Earth, oceans and animal species may have a fighting chance to survive and continue thriving, for centuries to come. If you are interested in learning Aqualead and would like to find a Master in your area, visit the contact section of the website aqualeadinstitute.org, or email: aqualead1(a)gmail.com

APPENDIX I:

The Aqualead Principles

1. The purpose of Aqualead energy is to salvage the Earth and restore the planet's natural state of balance.
2. Aqualead practitioners and Masters are people who have received training and the necessary attunement(s) in order to practise and teach Aqualead energy healing.
3. Aqualead sessions and classes are free of charge. Voluntary donations only may be accepted.
4. Aqualead supports trees, vegetation and wildlife; all living things have the right to live free and undisturbed in their own natural environment.
5. Aqualead supports conservation, recycling and sustainable agriculture.

APPENDIX II:

Twelve Practical Tips to Keep the Earth Healthy and Green

Recycle paper, plastics, non-organic waste and everything else.
Recycle old computers, electronic devices and used ink cartridges at computer or office supply stores; old batteries are recyclable in all major hardware outlets. Use rechargeable batteries and a charger; bring cloth reusable shopping bags to stores instead of taking plastic.

Compost food waste and other organic residue.
This is a great way to reduce kitchen waste and create soil for the garden. Some municipalities will collect composting materials.

Go Veg: replace animal proteins.
You can have veggie burgers, hot dogs, cakes, pies, ice cream and chocolate mousse, without having any animal products in them. There are tons of vegetarian and vegan recipe books available for easy and simple ideas; you can also get a free vegetarian/vegan starter kit from:

- peta.org/living/vegetarian-living/free-vegetarian-starter-kit.aspx
- vegankits.com

or here:

- oprah.com/packages/vegan-starter-kit.html

By eating low in the food chain, you reduce pollution, animal cruelty and the waste of water and grains used towards meat production; eating fish and eggs is not vegetarian.

Buy animal-free clothing, and cosmetics that were not tested on animals.
The PETA (People for the Ethical Treatment of Animals) site has a list you can download of companies that test their products on animals, and others that don't. You can check their website here: peta.org/living/beauty-and-personal-care/companies/default.aspx; the Physicians Committee for Responsible Medicine is also a great resource: pcrm.org

Support organic farmers: buy organic foods and produce.
By supporting pesticide-free foods, you promote safe and responsible farming, and protect bees and other insects that pollinate the plants. You also encourage organic farmers.

Grow your own herbs, fruits and vegetables – in pots, or in the ground.
Mint, lettuce, cherry tomatoes and strawberries are an all-time favourite; it's a great activity for kids.

Plant more trees, shrubs and perennials in the yard.
Plant a forest meadow on your property; the trees create shade and shelter, and will attract birds and butterflies.

Use public transportation or bicycles in cities.
You will help reduce traffic, noise and pollution, all at once.

Reduce electricity consumption by turning out lights, and turning off unused appliances.
If everyone reduces their electricity consumption on a daily basis, it makes a huge difference to the environment in the end.

Avoid using insecticides, herbicides and other chemicals in or around the house.
This will improve your overall health, prevent soil and water contamination, and protect animals, birds and insects.

Use natural and biodegradable bath and cleaning products.
White vinegar, tea tree oil and lemon juice make great ingredients for natural cleaning products. Visit treehugger.com for more ideas.

Help pick up trash and litter in the woods.
I am always amazed by what I find on the ground while hiking in nature, and what I pick up along the way (be sure to wear work gloves if you do this). River side clean-up projects are also a great community activity.

FURTHER READING

Bord, Janet. *Fairies: Real Encounters with Little People:* Dell Publishing, New York, 1997.

Briggs, Katharine. *A Dictionary of Fairies:* Penguin Books, London, 1976.

Emoto, Masaru. *The Hidden Messages in Water:* Beyond Words Publishing, Hillsboro, 2004.

Hall, Judy. *The Crystal Bible:* Godsfield Press, Alresford, 2003.

Lübeck, Petter & Rand. *The Spirit of Reiki:* Lotus Press, Twin Lakes, 2003.

Mac Manus, Dermot. *The Middle Kingdom: The Faerie World of Ireland:* Max Parrish & Co. Ltd., Buckinghamshire, 1959.

Moorey, Teresa. *The Fairy Bible:* Sterling Publishing, New York, 2008.

ABOUT THE AUTHOR

Sabine Blais was born in Ottawa, Canada in September 1971. She obtained her Bachelor's degrees in both French Literature and Philosophy at Ottawa University, between 1990 and 1995. The author has published *The Psychic's Guide, Volume I: An Introduction to Psychic Development* in 2005, and has produced the *Women of the Earth: Healing Oracle Deck* in 2006. She has been a Karuna Reiki Master since 2006 and is a certified Kundalini yoga teacher.

In 2006, the author left Canada for Buenos Aires, Argentina, where she lived for five years. While there, she inadvertently channeled a new energy healing modality called *Aqualead* in August 2008, and began teaching it all over Argentina. It is a new energy that heals water inside living beings and all over the planet. She returned to Canada in June 2011, in the Gatineau region, where she still teaches Aqualead, travels and writes.

In August 2013, Sabine founded her own publishing enterprise, as an outlet for her books and artwork, called *Silgerond Press*. She also paints, plays the violin and flute, and does healing work at the environmental level. She has been vegan for eight years, and remains involved in animal rights and environmental issues.

For more information about her publications, please visit Silgerond Press: Silgerond.blogspot.com. She is also the founder and director of the *International Centre of Aqualead*, a non-profit organization; for information about Aqualead and the Centre, which is based in Canada, visit: aqualeadinstitute.org.